The FIELD GUIDE TO PHYSICIAN CODING

FOURTH EDITION

Betsy Nicoletti, MS, CPC

Founder, CodingIntel.com

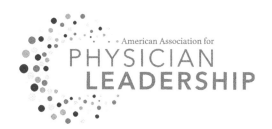

American Association for
PHYSICIAN
LEADERSHIP

AAPL books are available at special quantity discounts to use as premiums and sales promotions, or for use in corporate training programs. For more information, please write to Special Sales at journal@physicianleaders.org

This publication is designed to provide general information and is sold with the understanding that neither the author nor the publisher is engaged in rendering legal, accounting, ethical, or clinical advice. If legal or other expert advice is required, the services of a competent professional person should be sought.

13   8 7 6 5 4 3 2 1

Copyedited, typeset, indexed, and printed in the United States of America

PUBLISHER
Nancy Collins

EDITORIAL ASSISTANT
Jennifer Weiss

DESIGN & LAYOUT
Carter Publishing Studio

COPYEDITOR AND INDEXER
Robert Saigh

Table of Contents

Dedication

Colleagues and clients: I appreciate them both. Again and again, I turn to colleagues for answers beyond my knowledge, and they generously respond with their expertise and time. It allows me to be in a small consulting group (n=1) but have a much wider breadth in my scope of practice. Thank you to my clients who work with me year after year, asking me to audit services, educate providers and staff, and meet with them and their physicians.

BETSY NICOLETTI

About the Author

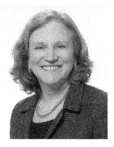

Betsy Nicoletti is an author, speaker and consultant. She developed The Accurate Coding System™ to help doctors get paid for the work they do. She simplifies complex coding rules for practitioners.

Betsy reads for a living: reads physician notes, that is. She is an experienced auditor and advises practices who are being scrutinized by their private payers or the government. She is an expert on E/M notes created by EMR systems.

She holds a Masters of Science in Organization and Management from Antioch, New England, and has worked in and around physician offices for over 25 years. She became a certified coder in 1999 and is a member of the National Speakers Association and the Medical Group Management Association.

In addition to this book, Betsy is the author of *Auditing Physician Services*, 3rd edition and *Everyday Medical Coding*, published by Greenbranch Publishing, and "Billing Guide to Preventive Medicine," a chapter in *Health Promotion and Disease Prevention in Clinical Practice*, 2nd edition, published by Lippincott, Williams and Wilkins. Her journal articles have appeared in The Journal of Medical Practice Management, Family Practice Management, and Physicians Practice. She blogs at nicolettinotes.com.

In 2017, she founded CodingIntel.com.

Betsy is a national speaker. She has spoken at conferences sponsored by Greenbranch Publishing, MGMA, DecisionHealth, AAFP and County Medical Societies.

www.betsynicoletti.com
Blog—nicolettinotes.com

Introduction

Hidden in plain sight. Many of the answers to coding questions are found in just a few places: the editorial comments in the CPT® book, and in the general guidelines of the ICD-10-CM manual, and in the Medicare Claims Processing Manual. Yet, they can be remarkably difficult to find. In this book, I help medical practice staff find answers to common, everyday coding questions. Each entry has a source citation. In addition to this book, two essential resources are the CPT® book and ICD-10-CM book. Read the editorial comments in the CPT® book about a code, and often, the question is answered.

Why do we care about coding in a fee-for-service environment and in the payment methods of the future? Because coding drives revenue and compliance. Even in new payment models of shared risk and savings, incentives and penalties are often based on fee-for-service coding. The Relative Value Units associated with a CPT® code are the current measure of physician work, for better or worse.

Coding is the process of assigning a procedure code (CPT® or HCPCS code) and a diagnosis code (ICD-10-CM) to a medical service that accurately describes what the physician or Non-Physician Practitioner did for or to the patient and the patient's condition or the reason for the service. It includes rules for the use of modifiers and description of multiple procedures.

Billing is the processes of sending a claim form or invoice to the patient or third-party payer for the service provided and collecting for those services.

Reimbursement is the payment for physician services and is dependent on government rules and policies, third party rules and policies, and mandated and associated fee schedules.

Purpose

The Field Guide to Physician Coding, Fourth Edition provides answers to common coding questions. I draw on definitions from the AMA and some coding and payment policies in use by Medicare and commercial payers. My goal in this book is to provide a resource that is quick and easy to use. The alphabetic format means a clinician, coder, or biller can quickly locate the topic and answer a question. Each topic entry follows a consistent format: definition, explanation, codes, coverage, billing and coding rules, key points, see also other entries, and citation. The citation is important for users who want more details or need to want to read the rules from the official source.

Topic selection

I included topics that come up over and over again in my work with medical practices. Over the course of a year, I meet with and speak to hundreds of physicians, nurse practitioners, and physician assistants, both one-on-one and in groups. Their questions serve as the basis for the topics in this book. It is a resource for my clients and for all of the other clinicians and coders and billers with whom I don't meet.

CPT° Companion

The Field Guide to Physician Coding, Fourth Edition will not replace your up-to-date copies of the CPT, HCPCS, and ICD-10-CM books. All offices must buy these resources yearly. You may need to refer to those resources as you read the answers in this book.

Collecting for physician services is hard work. I am constantly impressed with the dedication, knowledge and perseverance of physician office staff members, who do this job every day. I hope this book is helpful to you!

BETSY NICOLETTI

Advance Beneficiary Notice (ABN)

Definition:

An Advance Beneficiary Notice (ABN) is a written notification that a physician gives to a patient before providing a service notifying the patient that the service may not be covered or will not be covered by Medicare.

Explanation:

Medicare instituted the patient notification rules to protect their beneficiaries from financial liability when receiving a service that is not or may not be covered by Medicare. This written notice must be given to the patient prior to the patient's preparation for that service and must specifically inform the patient of the reason that the service may not or will not be covered. Practices cannot use blanket or blank ABNs.

Code: An ABN may be needed for many services.

Coverage:

ABNs are specific to Medicare although some third-party payers have similar limit of liability rules.

Billing and coding rules:

The first requirement for an ABN is to use the form approved by the Centers for Medicare and Medicaid Services (CMS). CMS revised the ABN form, and mandated the use of the new form starting March 1, 2009. Use form CMS-R-131 (03/11). Forms ABN-G and ABN-L are no longer valid.

A practice must execute the ABN properly prior to patient preparation for the service; the patient must not be asked to sign an ABN after being gowned and prepped to receive the service or after the service has commenced or the specimen has been drawn.

When completing the ABN, the specific name and description of the service must be listed. "Lab test:" is not specific. "CBC" is specific.

The reason that the practice believes the service may not be covered must also be specifically listed on the ABN. It is insufficient to write "Medicare may not cover this service." If the ABN is non-specific, such as "Medicare may not cover the service," the practice may not hold the patient financially responsible. Examples of specific reasons might be "Medicare does not pay for an electrocardiogram (EKG) for your condition" or "Medicare only pays for a pelvic exam every two years for a patient with no known risk factors, and your most recent pelvic exam was one year ago."

A family member can sign an ABN if the patient is unable to do so. If the patient refuses to sign the ABN but insists on receiving the service, a staff member should note this on the ABN and a second staff member should witness it.

CMS defines three events as the type that might trigger the need for an ABN. The first is the initiation of a new service, the second is for a reduction in the frequency of a service being provided to a patient, and the third occurs when a practice wants to terminate a service as non-covered but the patient wishes to continue to receive the service.

Medicare typically requires ABNs for procedures when the diagnoses are not listed as covered on either a National Coverage Determination (NCD) or a Local Coverage Determination (LCD), formerly known as Local Medical Review Policies (LMRPs). Healthcare procedures or services with an NCD or LCD have a list of indications for which the service is covered. If the patient's condition is not covered, then an ABN is needed.

An ABN establishes financial liability for a service. If a practice uses an ABN, it may hold the patient financially responsible for the service it is providing. Without it, the practice or lab providing the service cannot bill the patient if Medicare denies the claim. Medicare wants to make sure that the patient is making an informed decision about whether or not to receive the service, prior to receiving it.

The practice is required to keep the original of each ABN in the practice and give the patient a copy.

Related issues:

When submitting a claim to Medicare, there are four modifiers to indicate the status of that claim in relation to an ABN.

GA: Waiver of Liability Statement Issued as Required by Payer Policy" and should be used to report when a required ABN was issued for a service.

GX: "Notice of Liability Issued, Voluntary Under Payer Policy" and is to be used to report when a voluntary ABN was issued for a service.

GY: Item or service statutorily excluded or does not meet the definition of any Medicare benefit
GZ: Item or service expected to be denied as not reasonable or necessary. Using GZ tells the Medicare carrier no ABN is on file.

Understanding medical necessity as defined by an NCD or an LCD is key for use of ABNs. Use an ABN when those policies indicate that the patient's condition is not covered for that service or may not be covered. ABNs are not required for services that are never covered by Medicare; this includes cosmetic services and routine preventive services.

According to Medicare's manual instructions for ABNs, there are some situations that do not require ABNs. Here is what it says:

> ABNs are not required for care that is either statutorily excluded from coverage under Medicare (i.e., care that is never covered) or fails to meet a technical benefit requirement (i.e., lacks required certification). However, the ABN can be issued voluntarily in place of the Notice of Exclusion from Medicare Benefits (NEMB) for care that is never covered such as:
> - Care that fails to meet the definition of a Medicare benefit as defined in §1861 of the Social Security Act.
> - Care that is explicitly excluded from coverage under §1862 of the Social Security Act.
>
> Examples include:
> - Services for which there is no legal obligation to pay;
> - Services paid for by a government entity other than Medicare (this exclusion does not include services paid for by Medicaid on behalf of dual-eligible beneficiaries);
> - Services required as a result of war;
> - Personal comfort items;
> - Routine physicals and most screening tests;
> - Routine eye care;
> - Dental care; and
> - Routine foot care.

Key points:
- Use ABN form CMS-R-131.
- Execute the ABN prior to preparing the patient for the service.
- Describe the service specifically.
- Describe specifically the reason the service may not or will not be covered.
- Blanket ABNs are not legal.
- Blank ABNs are not legal.
- Submit with the appropriate GA, GX, GY, or GZ modifier.
- A practice may only hold patients financially responsible if they have properly executed an ABN.

See also: Medical necessity, local coverage determinations, national coverage determinations.

Citations:

ABN forms and information are available at http://www.cms.gov/Medicare/Medicare-General-Information/BNI/ABN.html

CMS, *Medicare Claims Processing Manual*, Pub 100-04, Chapter 30, Section 50, http://www.cms.gov/Regulations-and-Guidance/Guidance/Manuals/Downloads/clm104c30.pdf

Advance Care Planning

Definition:

According to the National Institute of Health, "An advance directive is a legal document that goes into effect *only* if you are incapacitated and unable to speak for yourself. This could be the result of disease or severe injury—no matter how old you are."[1] Advance Care Planning (ACP) is the process by which an individual indicates their medical wishes, if they should become unable to make those decisions in the future. There are two CPT® codes that describe the process of a health care professional discussing this with a patient.

Explanation:

CPT® developed Advance Care Planning codes in 2015, and in 2016, CMS changed the status indicator of these codes to active. That means, physicians and non-physician practitioners can bill and be paid for these discussions with patients, family members and surrogate care providers.

Codes:

There are two CPT® codes that describe ACP, 99497 and 99498. Both are time based codes. The second is an add-on code.

Coverage:

These are CPT® codes with a status indicator of active. Medicare has stated that it will cover these services for fee-for-service Medicare patients. Check with commercial carriers, Medicare replacement plans, Medicaid and Medicaid Managed Care.

Billing and coding rules:

This is the CPT® definition of ACP.

> CPT® code 99497 (Advance care planning including the explanation and discussion of advance directives such as standard forms (with completion of such forms, when performed), by the physician or other qualified health professional; first 30 minutes, face- to-face with the patient, family member(s) and/or surrogate); and an add-on CPT® code 99498 (Advance care planning including the explanation and discussion of advance directives such as standard forms (with completion of such forms, when

---

[1] https://www.nia.nih.gov/health/publication/advance-care-planning#what

performed), by the physician or other qualified health professional; each additional 30 minutes (List separately in addition to code for primary procedure))

The service is a face-to-face service, but may be between the provider and patient, the provider and family member or the patient's surrogate. This is an important shift in CMS policy. Usually, Medicare only pays for services that are face to face with the beneficiary. In this case, Medicare will pay for the physician for the non-physician practitioner to have a discussion about end-of-life planning and care with a family member or surrogate if that's more appropriate. This can be helpful when the patient is unable to participate in the discussion in a meaningful way. The service can be provided in the office or in a facility setting. This will be useful for physicians who are providing inpatient care. Often, the physician will see the patient and perform a hospital service in the early part of the day. If the patient's condition has worsened or changed, a family member may wish to speak to the physician about the type of care that the patient will receive. This family discussion for the purpose of making decisions about end-of-life care may be reported with ACP codes. This is not to say that updating family members or routine conversations with family members qualifies for reporting ACP.

This service may be reported on the same day as an Evaluation and Management (E/M) service, except for pediatric and adult critical care services. If this service is performed on the same day as an initial or subsequent wellness visit on a Medicare patient, the co-pay and deductible are waived. In that case, append modifier 33 to the wellness visit.

It isn't required that the healthcare professional complete forms at this visit. However, if forms are completed with the patient, the time of completing those advance directive forms maybe included in the ACP time.

CMS has not developed a national policy about this service. Individual Medicare administrative contractors (MACs) will develop their own policies. CMS has not instituted any frequency limitation on the service although individual MACs may do so. This service may be performed in the same month as transitional care management or chronic care management. Any specialty physicians may report the services, but a surgeon may not report the services during the global period.

Both Medicare and CPT® indicate that the services are the work of physicians and non-physician practitioners. A non-physician practitioner is an advanced practice nurse or physician assistant. Although CMS said that part of the service could be performed incident to and under the direct supervision of one of these billing providers, they cautioned that this work is provider work and should not be completely delegated to someone else.

These codes follow CPT® rules for determining time. That is, in order to bill for this service you must meet the threshold of over half of the stated time. You may report 99497 for services lasting 16 to 45 minutes. Use the add-on code 99498 if the time of the service is 46 minutes or more. The billing clinician must document time in the medical record.

Related issues:

This is one of the benefits that Medicare has initiated in support of primary care services. Although it is not limited to being performed by primary care clinicians, CMS expects that primary care doctors and other providers will provide the services.

Key points:

- Many clinicians discuss end-of-life care with patients. These codes provide the opportunity to be paid for the discussion.
- ACP is a time-based code. In order to reported the billing code clinician must spend 16 minutes in the discussion. Do not include the time of an office visit in this discussion.
- When the visit is performed on the same day as a Medicare wellness visit, the co-pay and deductible will be waived. That is, the patient will not have a patient due amount. Add modifier 33 to the ACP code.
- It is not required to fill out forms and order to bill for this service.
- The service requires a face-to-face encounter with the patient, the surrogate, or the family member.

See also: Wellness visits, Transitional Care Management

Citation:

https://www.cms.gov/Outreach-and-Education/Medicare-Learning-Network-MLN/
MLNProducts/Downloads/AdvanceCarePlanning.pdf

Anticoagulation Management

Definition:

Current Procedure Terminology (CPT®) developed two new codes for practices that manage patients on anticoagulation therapy. One is for teaching patients to use a home international normalized ratio (INR) monitor and the second is for non-face-to-face management of therapy.

Explanation:

These codes replaced deleted codes 99363 and 99364. Unlike the deleted codes, these codes have a status indicator of active and Medicare will pay them.

Codes:

93792: Patient/caregiver training for initiation of home international normalized ratio (INR) monitoring under the direction of a physician or other qualified healthcare professional, face-to-face, including use and care of the INR monitor, obtaining blood sample, instructions for reporting home INR test results, and documentation of patient's/caregiver's ability to perform testing and report results

93793: Anticoagulation management for patients taking warfarin, must include review and interpretation of a new home, office, or lab international normalized ratio (INR) test result, patient instructions, dosage adjustment (as needed), and scheduling of additional test (s) when performed

Coverage:

Fee-for-service Medicare will cover these services. They are active codes, and commercial payers will probably recognize and pay them.

Billing and coding rules:

93792 is used for educating patients who test their INR at home rather than going to the laboratory. Prior to starting this home testing, the patient needs to understand how do use the test reliably. This instruction and training is now a covered service. Notice that for patient/caregiver instruction and training, no work relative value units (RVUs) are assigned. Clinical staff or case managers would typically do this work.

93793 is payment for managing patients taking warfarin. It includes the review and interpretation of a lab test done in the home, office, or lab. This code does include work RVUs, recognizing that the physician/NPP must interpret the lab results. The work includes making a dosing adjustment if needed and scheduling additional tests, again if needed. The dosage does not need to be changed to report 93793. It is for a new test result.

Can these be performed on the same day as an Evaluation and Management (E/M) service? CPT® says a separately identifiable E/M service may be reported on the same day as 93792, instructions and training for a patient who will start home INR monitoring. CPT® says "Do not report 93793 on the same day as an E/M service." So, if the INR is done on the day of the visit and the physician/NPP interprets the result and gives the patient dosage instructions, do not report 93793 in addition to the E/M.

CPT® also states not to report either code during the service time of chronic care management (CCM) or transitional care management (TCM). (99487, 99489, 99490, 99495, 99496) During the service period would mean during any calendar month of reporting CCM and during the 30-day post-discharge period if billing TCM.

Related issues:

This is a non-face-to-face service paid by Medicare in recognition of the work primary care providers do that is not part of an office visit. Cardiology practices will also benefit from these codes.

Key points:

- Use 93792 only when the patient is starting on home INR monitoring. This is work the clinical staff does.
- A physician or NPP may bill for 93793 but not on the same day as an E/M service.

See also: Prolonged services: non-face-to-face

Citation:

CPT® 2018 Changes: An Insider's View

Assistant at Surgery Services

Definition:

Assistant at surgery services are services provided by a surgical assistant during a surgical procedure. Assistant at surgery services are payable by Medicare and other third parties for certain surgeries.

Explanation:

One of the indicators in the Medicare Physician Fee Schedule Database (MPFSDB) is for the assistant at surgery. Each CPT® and Healthcare Common Procedures Coding System (HCPCS) code in the MPFSDB has an assistant at surgery indicator. Here is the key to these four indicators.

0 = Payment restriction for assistants at surgery applies to this procedure unless supporting documentation is submitted to establish medical necessity.

1 = Statutory payment restriction for assistants at surgery applies to this procedure. Assistant at surgery may not be paid.

2 = Payment restriction for assistants at surgery does not apply to this procedure. Assistant at surgery may be paid.

9 = Concept does not apply.

Codes:

The modifiers used to report assistant at surgery services are:

80   Assistant surgeon

81   Minimum assistant surgeon

82   Assistant surgeon (when qualified resident surgeon not available). Modifier 82 is used in teaching facilities.

AS   Physician assistant, nurse practitioner, or clinical nurse specialist services for assistant at surgery

Coverage:

These indicators are in the MPFSDB but are typically followed by other third-party payers.

Billing and coding rules:

Bill the assistant at surgery services using the CPT® code billed by the primary surgeon and appending the appropriate modifier to the code.

Medicare allows 16% of the allowed amount for the primary surgery as payment for the assistant at surgery services if a physician is the assistant. Medicare applies the 85% payment rate to Physician Assistants and Nurse Practitioners who serve as assistants at surgery. That is, they pay 85% of 16 percent. Commercial payers typically pay between 20 and 25% of the allowed amount for the primary surgeon. It is common for practices to set their fee for their assistant at surgery services at 25% of the fee that they charge for their primary surgical services.

If the assistant at surgery indicator on the MPFSDB does not allow for an assistant at surgery, you are prohibited by Medicare from billing the patient for the service. Most third-party payer contracts also prohibit this. Most third-party payers follow the same assistant at surgery rules, although some have developed a different listing.

Related issues:

The condition of some patients may require an assistant at surgery, even for surgeries when this is not typically covered. A physician may bill for an assistant at surgery for surgery codes with a 0 indicator on the MPFSDB. The physician must document the medical necessity for this and send this documentation to the payer. This would include the patient's medical conditions, co-morbidity, or increased risk that necessitated the need for a surgical assistant.

Key points:

- Check the MPFSDB for the procedure and see if the assistant at surgery is allowed. If so, bill with a CPT® code of the primary surgeon, appending the appropriate modifier.
- If a Non-Physician Practitioner (NPP) provides the assistant at surgery care for a Medicare patient, use the AS modifier.
- When billing for a code with a zero indicator, which means that supporting documentation must be required for payment, be sure to indicate the reason that the assistant at surgeon was required for this service.

See also: Global surgical package, Medicare Physician Fee Schedule Database.

Citation:

CMS, *Medicare Claims Processing Manual*, Pub. 100–04, Chapter 12, Section 20.4.3, http://www.cms.gov/Manuals/IOM/list.asp

Care Management for Behavioral Health Conditions

Definition:

This 2018 Current Procedure Terminology (CPT®) code describes care coordination performed by clinical staff for patients with behavioral health conditions. In 2017, this service was reported with Healthcare Common Procedure Coding System (HCPCS) code G0507.

Explanation:

This code describes a service performed by a clinical staff member in caring for a patient with a behavioral disorder. No requirement exists that the clinical staff member be a behavioral health manager, which differentiates it from the psychiatric collaborative care model. Also, meeting the requirements for this code is easier than meeting the requirements for chronic care management.

Code:

99484: Care management services for behavioral health conditions, at least 20 minutes of clinical staff time, directed by a physician or other qualified health care professional, per calendar month, with the following required elements:

- initial assessment or follow-up monitoring, including the use of applicable validated rating scales
- behavioral health care planning in relation to behavioral/psychiatric health problems, including revision for patients who are not progressing or whose status changes
- facilitating and coordinating treatment such as psychotherapy, pharmacotherapy, counseling and/or psychiatric consultation
- continuity of care with a designated member of the care team

Coverage:

These are CPT® codes, with a status indicator of active. Original Medicare will pay for these. Check with Medicare Advantage and commercial payers.

Billing and coding rules:

To be eligible, patients must have an identified psychiatric or behavioral health condition that requires assessment, planning, and treatment. These conditions may be pre-existing or newly diagnosed. Patients may have other medical conditions, but this is not a requirement for the use of the code. The service is billed by the physician or non-physician practitioner (NPP) for the work done by clinical staff for a patient with behavioral health problems, including substance abuse. According to CPT®, a treatment plan must be in place. Documentation should include what was done.

The CPT® coding tip states that if the physician or other qualified health care professional (NPP) personally performs these activities, his or her time may be used to meet the 20-minute threshold as long as the time isn't counted toward another reimbursable service. That is, you can't get paid for the same service twice.

The reporting professional must have Evaluation and Management (E/M) services within his or her scope of practice. That limits the reporting of these services to physicians, nurse practitioners (NPs) and physician assistants (PAs). The service is reported and supervised by the physician or NPP, but the clinical staff does the work. Even if a licensed social worker is doing the work, do not use the social worker's National Provider Identifier (NPI) to report the service. This code may be reported in the same month as CCM as long as the practice is not double counting the time or services of one for the other. Code 99484 may not be reported in the same month as the psychiatric collaborative care codes, 99492, 99493, and 99494.

Time spent coordinating care if the patient is in the emergency department (ED) may be counted, but time may not be counted if the patient is an inpatient or in observation status.

The 20-minute threshold may be met by time spent by the physician/NPP or by the clinical staff under the direction of the physician/NPP. Unlike codes 99492, 99493, and 99494, the clinical staff member doing the work need not need be a behavioral health specialist or have qualifications to perform psychotherapy. However, if the professional is qualified to perform psychotherapy and provides that service, it may be billed during the same month as 99484. When the Centers for Medicare and Medicaid Services (CMS) initiated these as HCPCS codes in 2017, they said they were applying the term clinician in the same sense as CPT®: "We will apply the same definition of the term 'clinical staff' that we have applied for chronic care management (CCM) to G0507, namely, the CPT® definition of this term, subject to the incident to rules and regulations and applicable state law, licensure and scope of practice at 42 CFR 410.26. For G0507, then, we note that the term 'clinical staff' will encompass or include a psychiatric or other behavioral health specialist consultant, if the treating practitioner obtains consultative expertise." (Code G0507 in 2017 is 99484 in 2018.)

Related issues:

Many primary care practices provide care management services for patients with behavioral health diagnoses. Some may be able to meet the requirements of the collaborative care codes but many more will be able to document 20 minutes of case management, described by code 99484. Groups doing chronic care management can add this as a service for appropriate patients.

Key points:

- Lower payment than psychiatric collaborative care codes but fewer requirements
- May be performed by clinical staff; a behavioral health manager not required
- The service may be billed if the 20 minutes is performed personally by the physician or NPP
- A verbal consent is sufficient to start the service but must be obtained
- Requires an initial assessment, use of validated rating scales, (such as the depression scale,) behavioral health care planning and revisions to the plan, facilitating and coordinating treatment, such as psychotherapy medication management or psychiatric consultation if required, and continuity of care with the designated team member

See also: chronic care management, psychiatric collaborative care management

Citation:

CPT® 2018

Care Plan Oversight (CPO) – CPT® Codes (Non-Medicare)

Definition:

Care Plan Oversight (CPO) is a non–face-to-face service provided by a physician for a patient who requires complex, multi-disciplinary care. Medicare does not recognize these CPT® codes but developed HCPCS codes to describe covered CPO services for Medicare patients. The definition and requirements are different.

Explanation:

These codes are used by physicians to describe coordination of care for patients who are under the care of a home health agency (HHA) hospice, or in a skilled nursing facility (SNF). The patients must require complex supervision and management. Low intensity or infrequent supervision services are considered part of the pre and post work of face-to-face Evaluation and Management (E/M) services. These time-based codes are billed per calendar month.

Codes: 99374 to 99380.

Coverage:

These codes have Relative Value Units (RVUs) in the MPFSDB; however, they have a status indicator of bundled, and are not paid by Medicare. Many private payers, however, will pay them.

Billing and coding rules:

These codes are time-based codes described by the care the patient is receiving, (HHA, hospice, or SNF); and by time, 15 to 29 minutes or 30 minutes or more. Whenever time is used to select a CPT® code, time must be documented in the medical record as well as on the billing sheets.

Many practices find using log sheets useful to document this service if the practice is using a paper record. Each entry on the log sheet should include the date of service, a brief description of the nature of the supervision and the coordination, the amount of time spent on the patient, and the initials of the clinician providing the service.

The physician should document this information whenever supervision is performed.

At the end of the calendar month, if the threshold time of 15 minutes is met, bill for the service. These codes are for the work of the physician only and are not to be used for staff time. Nurses, medical assistants, or other employees of the physicians may not provide this service.

Only one physician should report this service in any calendar month for a particular patient.

The patient must require complex review of the care plan and condition, and this must require multiple phone calls, data review unrelated to an E/M service, and discussion with other healthcare providers.

The definition of these codes, unlike the Medicare HCPCS care plan oversight codes, allows the provider to bill for time spent discussing the patient's condition with family members, legal guardians, or other caregivers.

Related issues:

Most insurance companies will not pay for telephone calls, record review, or any non–face-to-face service time with a patient. Care plan oversight is one of the few covered services for a non–face-to-face service.

Key points:

- Use these codes for non-Medicare patients. Medicare uses HCPCS codes to describe services similar to these.
- Document time spent, what was done, and the dates the service was performed. Initial each entry and sign the log at the end of the month.
- Bill for a calendar month with a start and end date as the first and last date of the month.
- Include only provider time.
- Only one provider per month may bill for this service.
- Put the home health agency or hospice Unique Provider Identification Number on the claim form.

See also: Care plan oversight for Medicare patients.

Citation:

CMS, *Medicare Claims Processing Manual*, Pub 100–4, Chapter 12, Section 180, http://www.cms.gov/Manuals/IOM/list.asp

Care Plan Oversight for Medicare Patients

Definition:

Care Plan Oversight (CPO) is the supervision of a patient receiving Medicare-covered home health agency (HHA) or hospice services who requires supervision for complex and multi-disciplinary treatment.

Explanation:

Medicare developed these care plan services to pay physicians and NPPs for providing complex treatment supervision to patients who require coordination of multi-disciplinary care. It allows a provider to be paid for non–face-to-face services, when these services are greater than 30 minutes in a calendar month, the patient's condition is complex, and significant coordination of care is required.

Codes:

These services are defined and billed to Medicare using the following codes.

G0181: Physician supervision of a patient receiving Medicare-covered services provided by a participating home health agency (patient not present) requiring complex and multidisciplinary care modalities involving regular physician development and/or revision of care plans, review of subsequent reports of patient status, review of laboratory and other studies, communication (including telephone calls) with other healthcare professionals involved in the patient's care, integration of new information into the medical treatment plan and/or adjustment of medical therapy, within a calendar month, 30 minutes or more.

G0182: Physician supervision of a patient receiving Medicare-covered services provided by a participating Hospice (patient not present) requiring complex and multi-disciplinary care modalities involving regular physician development and/or revision of care plans, review of subsequent reports of patient status, review of laboratory and other studies, communication (including telephone calls) with other healthcare professionals involved in the patient's care, integration of new information into the medical treatment plan and/or adjustment of medical therapy, within a calendar month, 30 minutes or more.

Coverage:

Medicare beneficiaries. Check with commercial payers to see if they cover the CPT® CPO codes or the HCPCS codes.

Billing and coding rules:

The coding rules for this service are detailed and specific. Many physicians provide this service without ever billing for it.

Time spent in the coordination activities must be documented in the medical record, along with a brief description of the work performed, the date of the work, and the signature of the provider. The services must be provided by the same physician who certified the patient and signed the form for HHA or hospice services. A qualified NPP may provide CPO if that NPP has a collaborative agreement with the physician who signed the certification for HHA or hospice services.

The physician providing the service may not be an employee or director, paid or voluntary, of the HHA or hospice providing the care or have any significant financial arrangement with those organizations.

Only one physician in a month may provide and be paid for CPO. To bill for CPO, the physician must have seen the patient and billed for an E/M service within the last six months. The physician or NPP must provide 30 minutes of CPO in a calendar month.

In addition to receiving HHA or hospice service, the beneficiary must require complex, multi-disciplinary supervision to manage his or her care.

According to the Medicare claims processing manual, you can bill for CPO for time spent on the following activities:

- Regular physician development and/or revision of care plan
- Review of subsequent reports of patient's status
- Review of related or laboratory or other studies
- Communication with other healthcare professionals not employed in the same practice who are involved in the patient's care
- Integration of new information into the medical treatment plan
- Adjustment of medical therapy.

These activities below may not be counted in the time billed for CPO:

- Time spent discussing the patient's care with the physician's own staff member
- Time spent for any staff member activities
- Time spent in discussing the patient's care with the patient's family member or caregiver. This is a distinction between the Medicare defined HCPCS code and the CPT® definition of care plan oversight.
- The routine renewal of drug prescriptions
- The review of diagnostic test results related to an E/M service
- Travel time, time spent in submitting claims, or time spent calculating CPO time

- Time and work spent in providing discharge services, including 99217, 99238, and 99239
- Post-op care in the global period

Bill with the first and last calendar date of the month on the claim form and include the UPIN/NPI of the home health agency or hospice organization on your claim form.

The NPP may bill for CPO services, however, they may not certify the plan of care. The Internet Only Manual (IOM) Section 100-4, Chapter 12, Section 180, A: Home Health CPO states:

> "Non-Physician Practitioners can perform CPO services only if the physician signing the plan of care provides ongoing care under the same plan of care as does the NPP billing for CPO and either:
> - The physician and NPP are part of the same group practice; or
> - The NPP is a nurse practitioner or clinical nurse specialist, the physician signing the plan of care also has a collaborative agreement with the NPP; or
> - The NPP is a physician assistant, the physician signing the plan of care is also the physician who provides general supervision of physician assistant services for the practice.
>
> Billing may be made for care plan oversight services furnished by an NPP when:
> - The NPP providing the care plan oversight has seen and examined the patient;
> - The NPP providing the care plan oversight is not functioning as a consultant whose participation is limited to a single medical condition rather than multidisciplinary coordination of care; and
> - The NPP providing the care plan oversight integrates his or her care with that of the physician who signed the plan of care."

Related issues:

This is one of the few services allowing physicians to be paid for non–face-to-face time. Typically, time spent on phone calls, coordination of care, and record review are considered part of the pre-work and post work of Evaluation and Management services.

Key points:
- Document time, a brief description of the nature of the activity, and the date the service was performed. Sign the documentation.
- Patients receiving Medicare covered home health agency or hospice service are eligible for this benefit. Unlike the CPT® CPO codes, Medicare does not pay for CPO for patients in a skilled nursing facility.

- The patient must require supervision of complex multi-disciplinary care.
- Only one physician may bill for CPO time in a month. It must be the same physician who certified the patient for home health agency (HHA) or hospice care.
- An NPP may provide CPO services when the NPP has a collaborative agreement with the physician who certified the patient for home health agency care or hospice services.
- Review the list of services that may be included in time.
- Remember that the physician must have no financial arrangement with and may not be a voluntary director of the hospice or home health agency.

See also: Care plan oversight, CPT® codes, Transitional Care Management

Citation:

CMS, *Medicare Claims Processing Manual*, Pub 100-4, Chapter 12, Section 180, http://www.cms.gov/Manuals/IOM/list.asp

Category of Code Charts

OFFICE SERVICES			
In this place of service/ status of patient	**For this payer**	**Then**	**Use this category of code**
In the office, self-referred	For All Payers	➡	New or established patient 99201-99205, 99211-99215
In the office, consultation	If Medicare or Insurance doesn't recognize consults	➡	New or established patient 99201-99205, 99211-99215
	If Commercial	➡	Office/Outpatient Consultation 99241-99245

INPATIENT			
In this place of service/status of patient	**For this payer**	**Then**	**Use this category of code**
In the hospital, inpatient status—initial service by **admitting physician**	If Medicare or Insurance doesn't recognize consults	➡	Initial hospital service, 99221-99223 with AI modifier
	If Commercial	➡	Initial hospital service, 99221-99223 with no modifier
In the hospital, inpatient status **consultation**—first visit this admission	If Medicare or Insurance doesn't recognize consults	➡	Initial hospital service, 99221-99223 with no modifier
	If Commercial	➡	Inpatient consultation codes 99251-99255
In the hospital, inpatient status—follow up visit	For All Payers	➡	Subsequent hospital visits 99231-99233
	All Doctors		
In the hospital, inpatient status—discharge day by **admitting physician**	For All Payers	➡	Discharge code 99238 99239 (greater than 30 minutes)
In the hospital, inpatient status—discharge day by **consulting physician**	For All Payers	➡	Subsequent hospital visits 99231-99233
Surgery in the global period	For All Payers		No separate charge

EMERGENCY DEPARTMENT			
In this place of service/status of patient	**For this payer**	**Then**	**Use this category of code**
Emergency Department—**called to see own patient**	If Medicare or Insurance doesn't recognize consults	➡	Emergency Department visits 99281-99285
	If Commercial	➡	New or established patient 99201-99205, 99211-99215
Emergency Department—**in consultation**	If Medicare or Insurance doesn't recognize consults	➡	Emergency Department visits 99281-99285
	If Commercial	➡	Office/Outpatient Consultation 99241-99245

OBSERVATION			
In this place of service/ status of patient	**For this payer**	**Then**	**Use this category of code**
Patient in observation status, **admitting physician**—initial service	For All Payers	➡	Observation codes 99218-99220, 99234-99236 99234-99236—admit and discharge or same calendar date
Patient in observation status, **admitting physician**—subsequent visit	For All Payers	➡	Subsequent observation codes 99224-99226
Patient in observation status, **admitting physician**—discharge visit	For All Payers	➡	Observation discharge 99217
Patient in observation status, **consulting physician**—initial service	If Medicare or Insurance doesn't recognize consults	➡	New or established patient 99201-99205, 99211-99215
	If Commercial	➡	Office/Outpatient consultation 99241-99245
Patient in observation status, **consulting physician**— subsequent day	If Medicare or Insurance doesn't recognize consults	➡	Established patient 99211-99215
	If Commercial	➡	Subsequent observation codes 99224-99226
Patient in observation status, **consulting physician**— discharge day	If Medicare or Insurance doesn't recognize consults	➡	Established patient 99211-99215
	If Commercial	➡	Subsequent observation codes 99224-99226

Certification of Home Health Services

Definition:

Medicare pays physicians for the work required to plan and review Medicare-covered home health services for patients.

Explanation:

In 2001, Medicare added coverage to pay physicians for creating and reviewing care plans for patients receiving Medicare covered home health services. The initial certification may be billed once, when the patient has not received home health services in the past 60 days. The re-certification may be billed 60 days after the initial certification.

Codes:

G0179: Physician re-certification for Medicare-covered home health services under a home health plan of care (patient not present). This includes contacts with the home health agency and review of patient status reports required to affirm the initial implementation of the plan of care, per re-certification period.

G0180: Physician certification for Medicare-covered home health services under a home health plan of care (patient not present). This includes contacts with the home health agency and review of patient status reports required to affirm the initial implementation of the plan of care, per certification period.

Coverage:

Medicare beneficiaries receiving Medicare-covered home health services. Only a physician may bill for this service.

Billing and coding rules:

The physician who provides this service may not be an employee of the HHA or have a significant financial or contractual relationship with the home health agency.

Physicians must create and review the plan of care and the data collected by the HHA and maintain a record of this in their own medical record. The HHA may not simply prepare the plan for physician signature and maintain the certification in its own record.

Physician work that is related to and billed as care plan oversight must be separate and distinct from the work of this certification. CMS will not pay for the certification and care plan oversight for the same minutes in the month. A physician may provide and bill for an E/M service in the same month as the certification for home healthcare certification. The time spent in the home health certification should be distinct from the pre-work and post work of the visit, and from the visit itself.

Document in the physician's medical record the creation of the plan and the distinct work of the certification. For example, the plan for a progress note might include a discussion of the patient's need for home health services and a brief description of the plan of care. The physician's office should keep a copy of the certification and re-certification in its own chart, as well as documentation of phone calls and data review from the home health agency.

The plan of care should include the patient's diagnoses, the type of services, supplies and equipment that is required, the frequency of the visits ordered, prognosis, rehabilitation potential, functional limitations, activities permitted, nutritional requirements, medications and treatment, safety measures, and instructions for discharge.

NPPs may not bill for these services.

Unlike Care Plan Oversight (CPO), there is no minimum time spent in a calendar month to meet the requirements of this code. Physicians need to provide a face-to-face service with a patient prior to certifying them for home healthcare.

Starting January 1, 2011, a face-to-face visit with the patient is required prior to certification of home health. A Non-Physician Practitioner (NPP) may perform the face-to-face service if working in collaboration with a physician. This face-to-face encounter must be documented on the certification and must occur within 90 days prior to the start of home healthcare, or within 30 days after the start of the care. If the physician had seen the patient within the previous 90 days but the patient's condition had changed, requiring the order for home health, the physician must see the patient within 30 days of admission to home health.

Related issues:

Physicians are not typically paid for non–face-to-face services to patients. Billing for certification and re-certification of home health services and care plan oversight are two instances in which they can be paid. The billing and coding rules for each are specific and complex; however, the potential revenue will make it worthwhile for many physician practices to take the time to learn the rules.

Key points:
- Bill for G0179 for the initial home health services certification. It requires that the physician has had a face-to-face service with the patient 90 days prior to the certification or within 30 days.
- Bill G0180, the re-certification, after 60 days from the initial certification if the patient remains on home health services and the physician has reviewed the data collected by the home health agency and re-certified the need for the services.
- Physicians with significant financial or contractual arrangements with the home health agency may not bill for this service.
- Document phone calls, data review, and re-certification in the medical record.
- Don't double dip. Physicians cannot be paid for the same time in providing care plan oversight and certification. Both are billable in the same month if the work performed is distinct.

See also: Care plan oversight, care plan oversight for Medicare patients.

Citations:

Federal Register, Vol. 65, No. 212, Nov. 1, 2000, pp. 65406–65408.

http://www.cms.gov/Manuals/IOM/list.asp

Medicare General Information, Eligibility and Entitlement Manual, Chapter 4, Section 30

Medicare Claims Processing Manual, Pub 100-04, Chapter 12, Section 180.1

https://www.cms.gov/Outreach-and-Education/Medicare-Learning-Network-MLN/MLNMattersArticles/Downloads/SE1436.pdf

Cerumen Removal

Definition:

There are two CPT® codes for cerumen removal, one for lavage performed by clinical staff and one for removal with instrumentation, performed by a physician or NPP.

Explanation:

Many practices found that although they billed for cerumen removal at the time of an office visit or physical exam, the service was not paid by most of their payers. In July 2005, a standard definition of when to bill this service was published in the *CPT® Assistant* and agreed upon by the American Academy of Otolaryngology–Head and Neck Surgery (AAO–HNS).

Codes: 69209 and 69210.

Coverage:

Many payers bundled payments for cerumen removal into the E/M service, regardless of whether or not a 25 modifier was applied to the E/M service. Their claims editing system simply overrode that edit.

Billing and coding rules:

Bill 69209, removal impacted cerumen using irrigation/lavage, unilateral, when a clinical staff member performs this service. Although CPT® defines the service as unilateral, Medicare does not increase the payment when it is performed bilaterally.

To bill 69210, the following criteria must be met per CPT® and the AAO–HNS:

The service must be performed by the physician or NPP, not by a staff member. It is payable only if the cerumen is impacted and is removed with instrumentation, such as a microscope, curette, wire loops or suction. Lavage alone does not meet the criteria for using 69210. The cerumen should be considered impacted only if any one or more of the following are present:

- Visual considerations: Cerumen impairs exam of clinically significant portions of the external auditory canal, tympanic membrane, or middle ear condition.
- Qualitative considerations: Extremely hard, dry, irritative cerumen causes such symptoms as pain, itching, hearing loss, etc.

- Inflammatory considerations: The cerumen is associated with a foul odor, infection, or dermatitis.
- Quantitative considerations: The patient has an obstructive, copious cerumen that cannot be removed without magnification and multiple instrumentations requiring physician skills.

Starting in 2014, this code is no longer bilateral. Append modifier 50 if the service is performed bilaterally. However, Medicare does not pay additionally if it is done bilaterally.

Related issues:

A practice may not bill 69210 if a nurse provides this service. Use 69209 for ear lavage by a nurse.

Key points:

- Make sure that the documentation shows that one or more of the above characteristics are met.
- Remember that 69210 must be performed by a physician or Non-Physician Practitioner.
- For ear lavage, use 69209.
- If done on the same day as an E/M service, append modifier 25 to the E/M service. If payment is denied, be prepared to appeal, with the reference and documentation.

See also: Nurse visits.

Citation:

American Academy of Otolaryngology–Head and Neck Surgery, http://www.sccma-mcms.org/Portals/19/assets/docs/Coding%20Update%2069210.pdf

Chronic Care Management (CCM)

Definition:

Current Procedure Terminology (CPT®) has developed codes for the cognitive work of managing patients with serious chronic diseases that is not related to an Evaluation and Management (E/M) service. A physician or NPP supervises and the clinical staff performs this work.

Explanation:

The Centers for Medicare and Medicaid Services (CMS) and the American Medical Association (AMA) have increasingly sought to provide reimbursement for the cognitive work and coordinating of care for patients with significant, chronic diseases done by physicians and non-physician practitioners (NPPs) between visits.

Codes:

99487: Complex CCM services, with the following required elements:

- Multiple (two or more) chronic conditions expected to last at least 12 months or until the death of the patient
- Chronic conditions place the patient at significant risk of death, acute exacerbation/decompensation, or functional decline
- Establishment or substantial revision of a comprehensive care plan
- Moderate or high complexity medical decision making
- 60 minutes of clinical staff time directed by a physician or other qualified health care professional, per calendar month

+ 99489: each additional 30 minutes of clinical staff time directed by a physician or other qualified health care professional, per calendar month (List separately in addition to code for primary procedure.)

99490: Chronic care management services, at least 20 minutes of clinical staff time directed by a physician or other qualified health care professional, per calendar month, with the following required elements:

- Multiple (two or more) chronic conditions expected to last at least 12 months, or until the death of the patient
- Chronic conditions place the patient at significant risk of death, acute exacerbation/decompensation, or functional decline
- Comprehensive care plan established, implemented, revised, or monitored

Coverage:

These are active CPT® codes, but check with your commercial payers for coverage.

Billing and coding rules:

This is for the care provided by a physician or NPP and his or her clinical staff in a calendar month that is not part of a face-to-face visit. It requires the use of certified electronic health record (EHR). The patient must have 24-hour-a-day, 7-day-a-week access to address urgent needs, and this does not include an answering service informing the patient to go to the emergency department (ED). The patient must have access to continuity of care with a designated physician/NPP.

The service requires development of, revision of, and monitoring of a comprehensive care plan and the management of the plan. It includes coordination with home and community-based services, enhanced patient communication, such as email, and management of care transitions. Starting in 2017, the advanced consent need not be in writing, and faxing of the care plan to other team members is allowed. The patient must receive a copy of the care plan.

The care management for chronic conditions includes the following: systematic assessment of the patient's medical, functional, and psychosocial needs; system-based approaches to ensure timely receipt of all recommended preventive care services; medication reconciliation with review of adherence and potential interactions; and oversight of patient self-management of medications.

Although CMS recommends an initiating visit for established patients, it is not required. It is required for new patients, and it provides the opportunity for informed consent and development of the care plan. The initiating visit could be a welcome to Medicare visit, annual wellness visit, E/M service (codes 99212—99215), or the post-discharge service provided as part of Transitional Care Management.

If an initiating visit is performed, the physician or NPP may bill an add-on code (code G0506) once at the time of the initiating visit, starting January 2017.

+G0506: Comprehensive assessment of and care planning for patients requiring CCM services (List separately in addition to primary monthly care management service.):

- Billing practitioner personally performs extensive planning separate from the work of the E/M service or wellness visit
- Pays for the assessment and planning for CCM
- May only be billed once at the initiation of CCM

Related issues:

These services are for a calendar month. Bill on the date when the time threshold is met or at the end of the month.

CPT® and CMS have slightly different definitions of clinical staff. CMS stated in its 2017 Final Rule that, "Practitioners should consult the CPT® definition of the term 'clinical staff.'" Further, "If the billing practitioner provides the clinical staff services themselves, the time of the billing practitioner may be counted as clinical staff." CPT® defines a clinical staff member as "a person who works under the supervision of a physician or other qualified health care professional and who is allowed by law, regulation and facility policy to perform or assist in the performance of a specified professional service; but who does not individually report that professional service."

Key points:

- Requires care plan development for a chronically ill patient at an initiating visit (required for new patients, recommended for established patients)
- The initiating visit and an add-on code may be billed at the start of CCM
- Clinical staff, under the general supervision of a physician or NPP, provides and documents non-face-to-face care coordination during a calendar month
- Requires 24/7 access for urgent care needs
- Patient must consent to the service, and there is a patient due co-pay
- While typically non-face-to-face services, educational or motivational counseling may be provided face-to-face, and this may be included in the clinical staff time
- Time may never be counted twice to report two different services

See also: Psychiatric collaborative care management, care management for behavioral conditions

Citations:

CPT® 2018

https://www.cms.gov/Outreach-and-Education/Medicare-Learning-Network-MLN/MLNProducts/Downloads/ChronicCareManagement.pdf

CLIA Waived Tests

Definition:

The Clinical Laboratory Improvement Amendment (CLIA) of 1988 requires that all labs that test human specimens for diagnosis, prevention, or treatment be licensed by the Secretary of Health and Human Services. The amendment also identifies criteria for determining when a test is exempt from regulatory oversight and includes a list of these CLIA waived tests.

Explanation:

There are two types of CLIA-waived tests, those performed by a kit, and microscopy tests. CLIA-waived tests are typically simple and performed with manufacturer testing kits, which have little risk of error. Kit testing can be performed by a nurse or office assistant/tech with demonstrated competency in test quality control measures. Provider-performed microscopy (PPM) tests are performed on specimens that are not easily transferable and therefore need to be reviewed and read at the time of the patient's visit. Microscopy is a provider (physician) performed test.

Codes:

CMS provides a list of CLIA-waived tests on its web site. This listing includes the CPT® code and the description of each manufacturer's testing methodology.

Coverage:

These are covered services if the physician office is enrolled in the CLIA program and has a CLIA-waived test certificate.

Billing and coding rules:

CLIA-waived lab tests may be performed by physician's lab offices that are enrolled in the CLIA program, pay a biannual fee, and follow manufacturer instructions for the tests performed. PPM labs may be performed by medical practices, which are enrolled in this program and meet certain quality control and administrative requirements.

Related issues:

Some practices find that they are able to generate significant revenue doing a wider, more complex range of tests. To bill more than CLIA-waived tests, the practice must be licensed to do so.

Lab test reimbursement is not based on the Medicare Physician Fee Schedule Database (MPFSDB), but on the Medicare lab fee schedule. Lab services have an RVU value of 0 in the MPFSDB.

Key points:

- Enroll in the program and obtain a CLIA license.
- Look at the updated lists of CLIA-waived tests frequently.
- Perform the test in the approved manner.
- Assure that appropriate and timely quality control is being performed.
- Be sure that the test you are performing is being done using the method described in the CPT® book. For example, there are many ways to test glucose levels, so make sure that you select the CPT® code that corresponds with the method of testing you are using.
- Submit claims for CLIA-waived tests to CMS with the QW modifier.

See also: Medicare Physician Fee Schedule Database.

Citation:

CMS, http://www.cms.gov/clia

Cloning Notes in an Electronic Health Record

Definition:

Medicare Contractors and the Office of Inspector General (OIG) have raised concerns about excessive copying and pasting in medical record documentation in Electronic Health Records (EHRs). CMS has not released specific guidance about the topic, but the Office of Inspector General released two reports, with definitions, and asked CMS to develop a policy.

OIG definitions from their report:

Copy-Pasting. Copy-pasting, also known as cloning, enables users to select information from one source and replicate it in another location. When doctors, nurses, or other clinicians copy-paste information but fail to update it or ensure accuracy, inaccurate information may enter the patient's medical record and inappropriate charges may be billed to patients and third-party healthcare payers. Furthermore, inappropriate copy-pasting could facilitate attempts to inflate claims and duplicate or create fraudulent claims.

Overdocumentation. Overdocumentation is the practice of inserting false or irrelevant documentation to create the appearance of support for billing higher level services. Some EHR technologies auto-populate fields when using templates built into the system. Other systems generate extensive documentation on the basis of a single click of a checkbox, which if not appropriately edited by the provider may be inaccurate. Such features can produce information suggesting the practitioner performed more comprehensive services than were actually rendered.

Explanation:

An unfortunate outcome of EHRs is that physicians and NPPs must personally enter data either through typing, dictation, voice recognition or endless clicking. In response, many EHRs allow a clinician to carry forward large parts of a previous note. Physicians find it decreases typing to import sections of a previous note. As stated above, CMS has not developed a policy about this, but in response to the OIG report, has stated that it will develop a policy. Until then, practices must develop their own policies.

The Documentation Guidelines were developed in 1995 and 1997, long before most groups were using an EHR. These guidelines state that a review of systems (ROS) and past medical, family and social history taken at a previous encounter do not need to be re-recorded as long as there is evidence that the clinician reviewed them and updated them as needed. Those are the only two sections of an E/M note that the guidelines address. The history of the present illness is a description of the patient's symptoms or the status of the patient's conditions since last seen.

Codes:

This concept relates to both E/M codes and procedures although we think of E/M services as being most susceptible. Many EHR products have a feature that allows the user to import some or all of a previous note and edit it. Although this is convenient for the user, it raises questions about the accuracy of the record and the level of service reported.

History of the present illness (HPI):

The HPI describes the patient's symptoms or the status of their chronic diseases since last seen. These are new data. However, many clinicians find it helpful to copy a clinical summary from a previous note and update it as needed. Doing so saves the clinician time. Although this clinical summary usually starts the note, it isn't the HPI.

Example:

Clinical summary:

Pleasant 58-year-old with a past medical history of coronary artery disease, previous acute coronary syndrome. He had bypass surgery. His last cardiac catheterization was June 2011. At that time, bypass grafts were patent. The third obtuse marginal demonstrated 80 percent stenosis in the proximal third. The right coronary artery (RCA) demonstrated 100 percent proximal stenosis. The mid-RCA was supplied by collaterals. There was diffuse coronary disease. Ejection fraction was 55 percent. There was no intervention at that point in time.

HPI since last seen:

In November, he developed recurrent chest pain. He was ruled out for myocardial infarction and was discharged on metoprolol as well as imdur and he is no longer on Benicar. He has felt great over the past few months.

The ROS and past medical, family, and social history may be imported as long as the clinician notes it was reviewed and updated, or it was reviewed and no changes were required. If a complete ROS is documented at each visit, it gives the appearance of an overly templated note. Ask the clinician what the medical necessity is for that review at each follow-up.

The exam section should document only the exam elements performed at this date of service. Some clinicians want to import and edit a previous exam and state that it is no more or less accurate than starting with a template. Whichever method is used, the exam must reflect work at this date's visit. Use caution if the clinician uses the same exam for all presenting problems. If a comprehensive exam is documented at every visit, ask what the medical necessity is for that level of exam.

The assessment should only include problems and diagnoses addressed at this visit. Do not use the patient's entire problem list. The problem with copying an assessment and plan from a previous visit is that if not edited, it provides inaccurate clinical information.

Coverage: This is an issue for all payers.

Billing and coding rules:

CMS has a statement in the *Medicare Claims Processing Manual* that medical necessity and not the volume of documentation is the overarching criterion in selecting a level of E/M service. This does not directly address how the information was entered into the record. The OIG made specific recommendations in their two reports but does not develop policy.

Many organizations are developing policies. One physician colleague suggested the "The Golden Rule": The purpose of documentation is not to select a level of E/M service. Other healthcare professionals need to be able to treat the patient. The goal of this discussion is to protect the integrity of the medical record. When choosing an E/M level, the rule is that if you did not document it you did not do it so you cannot count it. With copying and pasting notes in EHRs, the rule is that you should not document it if you did not ask it, review it, examine it, or consider it. If you copied from a previous note, read your new note and see if it contains any details that do not meet one of those criteria. If so, delete that element.

Related issues:

See also E/M services.

Key points:

- Develop an internal policy with physician input
- The purpose of the medical record is clinical, not billing. It is critical to protect the integrity of the medical record

See also: Documentation Guidelines

Citations:

Office of Inspector General report "CMS and its contractors have adopted few program integrity practices to address vulnerabilities in EHRs", January 2014, OEI-01-11-00571

Office of Inspector General report "Not all recommended fraud safeguards have been implemented in hospital EHR technology" December 2013, OIE-01-11-00570

Cognitive Assessment and Care Plan Services

Definition:

In 2018, Current Procedure Terminology (CPT®) developed a code for physicians and non-physician practitioners (NPPs) to use when they assess a patient with cognitive impairment and they develop a treatment plan. This replaces Healthcare Common Procedure Coding System (HCPCS) Code G0505, which was active in 2017 and is now deleted.

Explanation:

This code is used when a physician or NPP assesses a patient with Alzheimer's disease or another cognitive impairment and develops a treatment plan for that patient.

Code:

99483: Assessment of and care planning for a patient with cognitive impairment, requiring an independent historian in the office or other outpatient, home or domiciliary or rest home, with all of the following required elements:

- Cognition-focused evaluation including a pertinent history and exam
- Medical decision making of moderate or high complexity
- Functional assessment (eg, basic and instrumental activities of daily living), including decision-making capacity
- Use of standardized instruments for staging of dementia (eg, functional assessment staging test (FAST), clinical dementia rating (CDR)
- Medication reconciliation and review for high-risk medications:
- Evaluation for neuropsychiatric and behavioral symptoms, including depression, including use of standardized instrument(s)
- Evaluation of safety (eg, home), including motor vehicle operation
- Identification of caregiver(s), caregiver knowledge, caregiver needs, social supports, and the willingness of caregiver to take on caregiving tasks
- Development, updating or revision, or review of an Advance Care Plan
- Creation of a written care plan, including initial plans to address any neuropsychiatric symptoms and referral to community resources as needed (eg, adult day programs, support groups); care plan shared with the patient and/or caregiver with initial education and support

Coverage:

These are CPT® codes, with a status indicator of active. Original Medicare will pay for these. Check with Medicare Advantage and commercial payers.

Billing and coding rules:

This code is used when the physician or NPP determines that a patient needs a comprehensive evaluation to establish or confirm a diagnosis, etiology, and severity for cognitive impairment. The assessment may be performed on a new or established patient. CPT® restricts billing the service more frequently than once every 180 days. The CPT® code describes this as a service for patients in the office/outpatient, home, domiciliary or rest home. It may not be provided in the nursing home or inpatient setting.

These services may not be reported on the same day as code 99483.	
Psychiatry services	
90785	Psychiatric complexity interactive
90791	Psychiatric diagnostic interview
90792	Psychiatric diagnostic interview with Evaluation and Management (E/M)
Testing/assessment	
96103	Psych testing
96120	Neuropsych testing
96127	Brief emotional behavioral assessment
E/M	
99201–99215	E/M office/outpatient services
99324–99337	Domiciliary rest home visits
99341–99350	Home visits
99366–99368	Team conferences (not paid by CMS)
99497–99498	Advanced Care Planning
These services may not be reported during the same time period as code 99483.	
99374	Care plan oversight (not paid by CMS) Per CMS, not CPT®
G0101	Care plan oversight
G0182	Care plan oversight
G0506	Initiating CCM visit

CPT® also indicates these may not be billed with code 99483.	
99487, 99489, 99490	Chronic care management (CCM)
99495–99496	Transitional care management (TCM)
99605–99607	Medication management by a pharmacist

CPT® has added an editorial comment in the 2018 CPT® book that code 99483 may not be reported with TCM or chronic care management (CCM). CMS did not have this edit in place, but I have added those codes above. Do not report 99483 with 99605, 99606, and 99607, CPT® codes for medication management provided by a pharmacist. These were not and are not covered services by Medicare and most payers. CPT® states not to report these with this cognitive assessment code, and I've included them in the chart above, payers will probably not recognize and pay them.

Code 99483 may be reported with prolonged services codes. Under the prolonged services, codes 99354 and 99355, CPT® notes that code 99483 may be reported with code 99354.

Keep in mind that time may never be double counted.

The service requirements are extensive, as you can see from the description above. But, with some planning and development of templates, it is a doable service. Many of the standardized instruments are already in use in the annual wellness exams. Staff members can administer these instruments.

Only clinicians who have Evaluation and Management (E/M) services within their scope of practice may perform these services. CMS describes these professionals as physicians and "eligible non-physician practitioners, such as nurse practitioners and physician assistants."[1] Psychologists, neuropsychologists and social workers may not bill 99483, because those professionals are not eligible to perform E/M services.

Related issues:

Although CMS discussed these codes in the section of the 2017 Final Rule devoted to increasing the accuracy of primary care payments, the codes may be used by physicians and NPPs in any specialty.

Key points:

- This code may only be used by a physician or NPP, who has E/M services within their scope of practice.

---

[1] 2017 Physician Fee Schedule Final Rule, page 318

- This assessment may not be done on the same day as an E/M service.
- Look at the requirements and develop a template that meets all the requirements for the code. Check with your specialty society for help.

See also: psychiatric collaborative care management, chronic care management

Citation:

CPT® 2018

Comprehensive Error Rate Testing (CERT)

Definition:

CMS's Comprehensive Error Rate Testing (CERT) program measures and reports the accuracy of paid fee-for-service Part A and Part B Medicare claims. The goal of the program is to reduce improper payments.

Explanation:

According to CMS, the CERT contractor randomly selects 40,000 claims for review for each reporting period. This review assesses each claim for the accuracy of the provider coding as well as the accuracy of the Medicare contractor's claims processing. This allows CMS to calculate a national improper payment rate, a contractor specific rate, and service-specific error rate. In addition, the CERT contractor assesses whether the claim complied with Medicare coverage, coding, and billing rules. The CERT contractor tracks the provider compliance error rate. CERT counts the following as errors:

1. Requests for which no documentation is received
2. Requests for which illegible or incomplete documentation is received
3. Errors in paid claims due to coverage, coding, or billing mistakes

These data are available for download from the CERT web site by Medicare Administrative Contractor and type of service. According to the CMS web site, the improper payment rate is not synonymous with a "fraud" rate.

Codes: All.

Coverage: Medicare.

Billing and coding rules:

If a physician office receives a request for medical record documentation for a specific service from the CERT contractor, the physician should carefully review the request and send the requested documentation. Sending this information is not a HIPAA violation. The practice does not need the beneficiary's signature to send the medical records, nor should the practice notify the beneficiary that the record was requested or sent.

The preferred method for submitting the data is via fax with a cover sheet that includes the bar code from the request. Even if mailed, the notes are scanned. If the legibility of the note is in question, faxing and scanning will certainly decrease its legibility. Be sure to send everything that relates to the service provided.

The patient name and another identifier should be on all pages sent. Sometimes the back page of a physician progress note in the office does not have the patient's name, so be sure to check for it.

If a provider fails to submit the requested documentation or if the claim was billed incorrectly, the provider will receive a request for a refund.

Respond to CERT requests promptly.

Related issues:

A CERT report provides important information about the error rate for each type of service paid by the Medicare Contractor. Although the claim volume for some services may be small for an individual contractor, in the aggregate, this is an excellent source of data. For example, established office visits have a significantly lower error rate than initial or subsequent hospital visits. Physician practices should review their own billing and coding and understand the coverage rules for services with a high error rate.

Key points:

- The CERT program measures the paid claims error rate nationally, by contractor, and by type of service.
- Physician overpayment errors will result in a request for a refund.
- Respond promptly to requests from the CERT contractor for medical record documentation. Sending medical records does not violate HIPAA regulations. A provider need not inform the beneficiary that a record was sent.
- Contractors will pay physicians who under-billed for services when these errors are discovered during CERT review.

Citations:

CMS, http://www.cms.gov/CERT

CERT Provider web site, https://www.certprovider.com/

https://www.cms.gov/Research-Statistics-Data-and-Systems/Monitoring-Programs/Medicare-FFS-Compliance-Programs/CERT/index.html

Consolidated Nursing Home Billing

Definition:
Consolidated nursing home billing is a Medicare payment method that includes payment for some Part B services in the payments made to the skilled nursing facility (SNF) when the patient is in a covered Part A stay.

Explanation:
The Balanced Budget Act of 1997 requires Medicare to pay for services for patients in a Part A stay with a single payment to the SNF unless the services are specifically excluded from the inclusive payment. This includes payment for some services performed by physicians that would typically be paid on a fee for service basis by Part B.

During the Part A stay, if a physician provides certain services such as the technical component of a diagnostic test that is included in the bundled prospective payment to the SNF, the physician must bill the SNF—and not Medicare or the patient—for that service (some exceptions apply). Other services performed by the physician or NPP after the Part A stay has ended must be billed to the SNF, and the SNF must look to the contractor for payment.

Some medications are included in the SNF consolidated payment, and some may be billed separately.

These rules apply to patients in a Part A covered stay whether they are seen in the SNF, the physician office, or an outpatient department. CMS updates the list of services included or excluded quarterly on its web site.

Codes: Vary by quarter.

Coverage: Medicare.

Billing and coding rules:
According to the CMS web site, the following services are separately payable during a Part A covered stay:
- Physician's professional services
- Certain dialysis-related services, including covered ambulance transportation to obtain the dialysis services
- Certain ambulance services, including ambulance services that transport the beneficiary to the SNF initially, ambulance services that transport the beneficiary from the SNF at the end of the stay (other than in situations involving transfer to another SNF), and roundtrip ambulance services furnished during the stay that transport the beneficiary offsite temporarily

to receive dialysis, or to receive certain types of intensive or emergency outpatient hospital services

- Erythropoietin for certain dialysis patients
- Certain chemotherapy drugs
- Certain chemotherapy administration services
- Radioisotope services
- Customized prosthetic devices

For Medicare beneficiaries in a non-covered stay, only therapy services are subject to consolidated billing. All other covered SNF services for these beneficiaries can be separately billed to and paid by the Medicare contractor.

When CMS states on its web site that the services listed above are separately payable, they mean the physician office may report these on a CMS 1500 form to Part B. Other services (such as the technical component of an x-ray or EKG) that are performed in any location for a patient who is in a covered Part A stay must be billed to the SNF and not to Medicare. This can be difficult for medical practices if a patient presents to the physician office during a covered Part A stay.

Related issues:

Consolidated billing covers patients in a Part A covered stay. For patients in a Part B covered stay, only the physical and occupational therapy provisions apply. Practices need to know the status of the patient to know whether to bill place of service (POS) 31 (skilled nursing facility) or POS 32 (nursing home) when they bill for physician services.

Key points:

- The professional component (E/M services, diagnostic test interpretation) of physician services may be billed to Part B for patients in a covered Part A stay.
- These rules apply whether the physician provides the service in the SNF, in their own office, or in the outpatient department.
- Check the excluded/included list quarterly if you provide these services.

See also: Nursing facility visits.

Citation:

https://www.cms.gov/Medicare/Billing/SNFConsolidatedBilling/index.html

Consultations

Definition:

An inpatient or outpatient consultation is a service provided by a physician or qualified NPP for the purpose of obtaining an opinion or advice regarding evaluation and treatment of a patient at the request of another physician or NPP. It is distinguished from another E/M service by the request for the opinion or evaluation, and requires that a report is returned to the requesting provider. If a transfer of care occurs, the service does not qualify as a consult, per CPT® in 2010. As of January 1, 2010, Medicare stopped recognizing the consultation codes. Commercial payers are free to recognize consult codes or follow Medicare's policy. CPT® defines consults as "a type of Evaluation and Management service provided at the request of another physician or appropriate source to either recommend care for a specific condition or problem or to determine whether to accept responsibility for ongoing management of the patient's entire care or for the are of a specific condition or problem."

Explanation:

A consult requires a request for opinion from another healthcare provider. The request must be documented in the patient's medical records. After the consultant sees and evaluates the patient, a report must be returned to the requesting provider.

CMS stopped recognizing consults as of January 1, 2010, because they believed there was a high error rate in the use of these codes. Consultation codes have higher Relative Value Units (RVUs), i.e., payment, than other E/M codes.

Codes:

99241–99245 for office, ED, observation and outpatient consults
99251–99255 for inpatient and nursing facility consults

Coverage:

Consultations are covered when medically necessary and the criteria for consultation are met. Fee-for-service Medicare no longer recognizes these codes, and many Medicare Advantage policies followed suit. Some commercial payers have stop recognizing these codes.

Billing and coding rules:

Consultation codes do not have new or established patient designations. A physician or NPP may bill a consult on a patient who is new or established to them, as long as the criteria for a consultation are met.

Who may request a consult? According to the CPT® definition, it may be another healthcare professional "or other appropriate source." However, since most payers require the NPI number of the requesting provider on the claim form, the requesting provider for a consult is a healthcare professional who has a provider number and is able to bill third parties on their own. This means patients referred to the practice by a friend who is a nurse, by a physician referral service, or who come on their own are not consultations, but are new or established patient visits.

In 2010, CPT® added in the concept of transfer of care to the definition of consults. Previously, the concept of transfer of care was only a Medicare concept. However, CPT® included this in their definition in the CPT® book in 2010. CPT® does say, however, that if the purpose of the visit is to determine whether to accept the care of the patient, a consult may be billed. If the patient's care is transferred, a new or established patient visit should be billed, not consultation visits. A complete transfer of care occurs when the physician or NPP requests that another physician or NPP take over complete care of the patient for the condition and does not expect to continue caring for that patient for that condition. This transfer of care might occur between two physicians of the same specialty, when a patient is sent between sub specialists or if a patient moves from one city to another and the care is transferred to another physician. The difference is that the referring physician will not continue treating that patient for that problem, but is transferring care to the second physician.

How must the request for consultation come to the consultant's office? The request may be in writing or verbal between the two clinicians. For example, an internist sees a patient with persistent elbow pain. The internist has tried conservative treatment, such as medicine, physical therapy and home exercises but the patient continues to complain of pain. The internist sees the patient on September 5, 2014, and suggests that the patient be evaluated by an orthopedist for the problem. The medical record in the internist's office on that date of service should indicate the request for an orthopedic consult. When the patient is seen by the orthopedist, the orthopedist should indicate in the consult report that the patient is being seen at the request of Dr. Internist.

Consultants may initiate treatment or order tests and still bill for a consultation. After evaluating the patient, the consultant must send a report to the requesting provider.

A physician or NPP may request a consultation from another member of their own group if that provider has specific expertise required for the patient's care that is beyond his or her own expertise. Neither supervision or transfer of care qualify as consults.

Consultations may be billed using time as the determining factor if more than 50% of the visit is spent in counseling, the nature of the counseling is described and the consultant documents the total time and that more than 50% of the total time was spent in counseling.

What codes should a physician use when billing a Medicare patient for a consult after 2010? In the office, bill a new or established patient visit. (Remember, a new problem does not indicate a new patient. A new patient is a patient who has never been seen by that physician or another physician of the same specialty in the same group in the past three years.) If the patient is in observation status, use new or established patient visit codes (99201–99205). If the physician is called to the Emergency Department (ED) to perform a consult, use the ED codes, 99281–99285 for Medicare patients. CPT® instructs a physician to use the office and outpatient codes in that situation, but Medicare wants the ED codes.

If the patient is an inpatient in the hospital, bill for the consultation using the initial hospital services codes, 99221–99223, commonly described as admission codes. These initial hospital services codes are not defined as new or established, and may be billed by the consulting physician on new or established patients. The consultant bills these codes for the first visit and bills for follow-up services with subsequent hospital visits. The admitting physician uses these same codes with an AI modifier, and that is how the payer distinguishes these services from the services of consulting physicians. AI is a HCPCS modifier that means, "principle physician or record."

Related issues:

Practices must watch their payers' web sites and newsletters to be sure that the payer still recognizes and pays for consultations.

Medicare as a secondary payer presents its own challenges.

Options for office "consults":

- Bill primary with consult codes. Will cross electronically to Medicare and be denied. Resubmit electronically, with a note in *other information* field about primary payment. Requires handling of every claim. If primary allowance is more than Medicare, and small secondary Medicare balance may be okay.
- Bill primary with new or established patient visit code. Will cross electronically to Medicare and be paid automatically. Less revenue. No extra handling of claim.

Options for hospital "consults":

- Bill primary with consult codes. Will cross electronically to Medicare and be denied. Resubmit electronically, with a note in *other information* field about primary payment. Bill primary with initial hospital services codes. How will they process multiple initial hospital services codes from different physicians?

Key points:

- Document the request for consultation in the patient's medical record. Many offices ask for a copy of the note for that date or ask the requesting provider to send you a written request for the consult.
- Document a verbal request in the consultation note (e.g., "I am seeing this patient at the request of Dr. Jones. In a phone conversation, he asked for my opinion about . . .").
- Document the written request ("I am seeing the patient at the written request of Dr. Jones for my evaluation of . . .").
- After performing the evaluation, send a report back to the requesting provider and keep a record that the report was returned.

See also: Shared visits, Incident to services, Time-based codes, Category of code charts

Citations:

Medicare Claims Processing Manual, Pub 100-4, Chapter 12, Sections 30.6.10 and 30.6.11, http://www.cms.hhs.gov/Manuals/IOM/list.asp

CMS, Transmittal 782, Change Request 4215, released December 16, 2005.

CMS, *MLN Matters,* issue 4215, December 20, 2005, updated February 25, 2013.

Critical Care Services

Definition:

Critical care services are health care services provided to a critically ill patient and are billed based on time documented in the medical record. The patient's condition must be critical, and the physician must provide intensive medical services to the patient.

Explanation:

The *Medicare Claims Processing Manual* describes the service in Chapter 12, Section 30.6.12 A:

"Critical care is defined as the direct delivery by a physician(s) medical care for a critically ill or critically injured patient. A critical illness or injury acutely impairs one or more vital organ systems such that there is a high probability of imminent or life threatening deterioration in the patient's condition.

Critical care involves high complexity decision making to assess, manipulate, and support vital system functions(s) to treat single or multiple vital organ system failure and/or to prevent further life threatening deterioration of the patient's condition.

Examples of vital organ system failure include, but are not limited to: central nervous system failure, circulatory failure, shock, renal, hepatic, metabolic, and/or respiratory failure. Although critical care typically requires interpretation of multiple physiologic parameters and/or application of advanced technology(s), critical care may be provided in life threatening situations when these elements are not present."

Codes: 99291 and 99292.

Coverage: Critical care services are covered when medically necessary.

Billing and coding rules:

When billing for critical care services, the patient's condition must be critical as described in the paragraph above, the physician must be providing treatment for the patient's condition, and the time spent in providing the critical care must be documented in the patient's medical record. Although these patients are usually located in the intensive care unit, location is not the driving factor in billing for critical care. Patients who are receiving critical care may be on a medical surgical floor or in the emergency department (ED). Conversely, simply because the patient is in the critical care unit does not mean that a physician can automatically bill for critical care.

The physician must be in attendance caring for the patient, meaning that the physician is on the unit, immediately available to the patient, and not caring for any other patient at that same time. The *Medicare Claims Processing Manual* describes this as "devoting his or her full attention" to the patient being treated. The physician may not include time spent on the phone directing the patient's care if he or she is off the unit during that time.

Time spent in critical care must be documented in the medical record. If time is not documented, the visit must be billed as a subsequent hospital visit. Physicians are paid much more for critical care than for subsequent hospital visits. Time is on your side but only if you document the critical care time. If the physician spends less than 30 minutes providing critical care service, bill the Evaluation and Management (E/M) service that is in the correct category (subsequent hospital visit, emergency department visit, etc.).

If a physician sees a patient multiple times on one date, add up the time spent during all visits per calendar date and bill that time. Physicians of the same specialty in a group should bill and be paid as if they were one physician. For critical care, this means the first doctor bills using code 99291, and all of the partners who see that patient and provide critical care on that date bill use code 99292, the add-on code. More than one physician can not bill code 99291 on the same date when the physicians are of the same specialty and in the same group. However, one physician must meet the entire time requirement for code 99291 before a partner can use code 99292.

Non-physician practitioners (NPPs) may provide critical care services if they are within their scope of practice. CMS states, however, that the time of a physician and an NPP may not be added together. That is, critical care may not be a shared service of the physician and NPP. This is a CMS rule, not a CPT® rule. Here is the citation from the CMS manual:

> "Critical care services may be provided by qualified NPPs and reported for payment under the NPP's National Provider Identifier (NPI) when the services meet the definition and requirements of critical care services in Sections A and B. The provision of critical care services must be within the scope of practice and licensure requirements for the State in which the qualified NPP practices and provides the service(s). Collaboration, physician supervision, and billing requirements must also be met. A physician assistant shall meet the general physician supervision requirements."

The chart (below) from the *Medicare Claims Processing Manual* shows how to use the codes, based on time spent providing critical care.

Total Duration of Critical Care 9292 x 4	Code(s)
Less than 30 minutes	99232 or 99233
30–74 minutes	99291 x 1
75–104 minutes	99291 x 1 and 99292 x 1
105–134 minutes	99291 x 1 and 99292 x 2
135–164 minutes	99291 x 1 and 99292 x 3
165–194 minutes	99291 x 1 and 9

Include time spent in the following services as part of critical care billing:
- Providing service at the patient's bedside
- Discussing the patient's condition with other physicians or other members of the patient's care team when on the unit and immediately available to the patient
- Reviewing data related to the patient
- Performing procedures bundled into the payment of critical care (listed below)
- Discussions with the family ONLY IF the discussion with the family involves obtaining clinically relevant history that the patient is unable to give or discussion with the family required because a family member must make medical decisions for the patient
- Writing notes in the chart

Do not include time spent in the following activities in your critical care time:
- Time off the unit, discussing the patient or giving orders by phone
- Discussions with the patient's family for the purpose of informing them about the patient's condition
- Performing procedures not bundled into critical care services
- Providing services to any other patients

The *Medicare Claims Processing Manual* specifically describes the need to document time:

The duration of critical care time to be reported is the time the physician spent working on the critical care patient's case, whether that time was spent at the immediate bedside or elsewhere on the unit and the physician remained immediately available to the patient.

Certain services are bundled into the provision of critical care. Include the time spent in providing these services in the total critical care time, but do not bill these services in addition to critical care:

- Interpretation of cardiac output measurements (CPT® 93561, 93562)
- Obtaining chest X-rays (71045, 71046)
- Drawing blood for specimen (HCPCS G0001) (CPT® 36415)
- Reviewing stored data in computers (e.g., ECGs, blood pressures, blood gasses, and hematologic data) (99090)
- Performing gastric intubation (91105, 43752)
- Performing pulse oximetry (94760, 94761 94762)
- Providing temporary transvenous pacing (92953)
- Managing ventilator settings (94002–94004, 94660, 94662)
- Doing peripheral vascular access procedures (36000, 36410, 36415, 36660)

If the physician performs other procedures, those may be billed separately. Do not include the time spent in performing nonbundled procedures into critical care time.

Can a physician be paid for another E/M service on the same day as critical care? Sometimes. The same physician may not be paid for an ED visit and a critical care service on the same day. A physician can be paid for an initial hospital service and a critical care service or can be paid for a subsequent hospital visit and a critical care service if the documentation shows the visits were **separate, distinct, medically necessary services**. Typically, the patient's status changes. For example, a physician may admit a patient in the morning to a medical unit. Later that day, the patient's condition worsens, and the patient is moved to critical care. The physician may bill for the initial hospital service and the critical care service as long as both are documented. (Remember, time must be documented in the medical record, not just the billing record, for critical care time.) Submit the bill with a modifier 25 on the initial hospital service, and send notes. A physician may bill for a subsequent hospital service and critical care, just as in the example above, if the patient's condition changes and both services are provided.

Medicare will only pay for critical care in the preoperative or postoperative period in addition to the global fee if the critical care is unrelated to the surgery. The *Medicare Claims Processing Manual* gives this billing advice about billing for preoperative critical care services:

"Preoperative critical care and/or postoperative care may be paid in addition to a global fee if the patient is critically ill and requires the full attention of the physician, and the critical care is unrelated to the specific anatomic injury or general surgical procedure performed. Such patients may meet the definition of being critically ill and criteria for conditions where there is a high probability of imminent or life threatening deterioration in the patient's condition.

- For preoperative care modifier 25 (significant, separately identifiable Evaluation and Management services by the same physician on the day of the procedure) must be used with the HCPCS code
- For postoperative care modifier 24 (unrelated Evaluation and Management service by the same physician during a postoperative period) must be used with the HCPCS code.

In addition, for each preoperative and postoperative care the diagnosis must clearly indicate that the critical care was unrelated to the surgery."

The manual instructs us to append modifier 24 on critical care provided on the same day as a surgery but after the procedure was performed and only when the critical care was unrelated to the surgery. Only one physician may be paid for providing critical care at any one time. If two physicians are attending to a patient in the same period, only one may bill if the patient is a *Medicare* patient.

Other third-party insurance companies may follow CPT® rules, which allows the physician to bill for complications of surgery.

Related issues:

Initial and subsequent hospital visits are per day codes. Critical care allows a physician to be paid for multiple episodes of care on a single day.

Key points:

- Document total critical care time per calendar date in the medical record.
- The patient must be critically ill and receiving treatment.
- Review the activities that can and cannot be counted in critical care time.

See also: Hospital discharge services, hospital initial services, hospital subsequent services, time based billing.

Citation:

CMS, *Medicare Claims Processing Manual*, Pub. 100–04, Chapter 12, Section 30.6.12, http://www.cms.hhs.gov/Manuals/IOM/list.asp

Diagnosis Coding

Definition:

CPT® and HCPCS codes tell the payer what was done. A modifier explains any special circumstances. The diagnosis code establishes the medical necessity for the service, telling the payer the reason for the service.

Explanation:

Claims for services provided after October 1, 2015 must use ICD-10-CM codes. Although the code sets are entirely different, the instructions to use these codes are similar for physician services. Hospitals use both ICD-10 diagnosis and procedure codes, but physician practices will use CPT® procedure codes and ICD-10-CM diagnosis codes.

The documentation guidelines tell providers of healthcare services that each service requires an assessment:

The documentation of each patient encounter should include:

- Reason for the encounter and relevant history, physical examination findings, and prior diagnostic test results;
- Assessment, clinical impression, or diagnosis;

And

- The CPT® and ICD-10-CM codes reported on the health insurance claim form or billing statement should be supported by the documentation in the medical record.

CMS Coding and Reporting Guidelines for diagnosis coding:

1. Use the ICD-10-CM codes that describe the patient's diagnosis, symptom, complaint, condition, or problem.
2. Use the ICD-10-CM code that is chiefly responsible for the item or service provided.
3. Assign codes to the highest level of specificity.
4. Do not code suspected diagnoses in the outpatient setting. Code only the diagnosis symptom, complaint, condition, or problem reported. Medical records, not claim forms, should reflect that the services were provided for "rule out" purposes.
5. Code a chronic condition as often as applicable to the patient's treatment.
6. Code all documented conditions which coexist at the time of the visit that require or affect patient care or treatment. (Do not code conditions which no longer exist)

In fee-for-service medicine, the fee is dependent on the HCPCS or CPT® code, and the diagnosis code validates the medical necessity but doesn't affect the amount of the payment. However, many groups are entering into contracts with risk adjustment for the acuity of the patient population. Medicare shared savings programs also use diagnosis coding to adjust end-of-year payments. Physician practices that are part of these Accountable Care Organizations should pay increased attention to the specificity, accuracy, and completeness of their diagnosis coding.

Codes:

ICD-10-CM codes are listed in the ICD-10-CM book and the Coding Clinic's quarterly update. The clinical modification version of the World Health Organizations code set is made by the Center for Disease Control and Prevention (CDC) and the American Hospital Association (AHA).

Coverage: All payers.

Billing and coding rules:

The explanatory material in the ICD-10-CM book provides specific rules for selecting a diagnosis code. These codes, adopted by all payers, are supplemented by payer rules that govern the ordering of codes and their use with certain diagnostic tests.

The ICD-10-CM book is divided into volumes: The first is a tabular list of diagnoses, and volume two is an alphabetical index. The user should look for a code in the index and then turn to the tabular list to select the most accurate and specific code. Never code from the alphabetic index.

In a physician note, diagnosis code information is written in the history as signs and symptoms, the reason for the visit, co-morbidities; and in the assessment. Code known diagnoses first. Code signs and symptoms if the diagnosis is not known. Each service provided should have a diagnosis code.

Clinicians using EHR are selecting their own diagnosis codes. This is often a source of intense frustration because the terms they use to search are not always found in ICD-10-CM descriptions.

Related issues:

How many diagnostic codes should a physician or NPP include on a claim form? The newest version of the CMS-1500 claim form allows for 12 diagnosis codes per line item.

Key points:

- Code for problems addressed at the current visit or service.

- Do not code past medical history or resolved problems when not addressed at that visit.
- If the diagnosis code is not known, code the signs and symptoms. However, once the diagnosis code is known, do not unbundle the diagnosis into signs and symptoms. It would be incorrect to give the patient the diagnosis of fatigue when the provider knows that it is a symptom of that patient's depression.
- Do not code rule-out or probable diagnoses in physician office coding. It is incorrect to code rule-out lung cancer. If that is an unconfirmed diagnosis, code shortness of breath or coughing up blood for the reason for the visit.
- Code to the highest degree of specificity.
- The ICD-10-CM code indicates certain codes that may not be used as primary diagnoses. Use these only in the secondary position.
- Code specific diagnoses when known in favor of non-specific diagnoses.
- Code the primary diagnosis first. You can code secondary tertiary or more diagnoses if addressed at that visit.

See also: Medical necessity, ICD-10-CM

Citations:

Introductory pages of ICD-10 book

CMS, *Medicare Claims Processing Manual*, Pub 100-04, Chapter 23;

http://www.cms.gov/Manuals/IOM/list.asp

www.cms.gov/Medicare/Coding/ICD10

Documentation Guidelines

Definition:

The Documentation Guidelines are a set of guidelines jointly prepared by CMS and the American Medical Association (AMA) that describe principles of medical record documentation.

Explanation:

The Documentation Guidelines serve as the basis of standards for E/M service documentation requirements. Good documentation is critical not only for patient care, but to ensure that payers have the information necessary to validate each claim.

These guidelines include general principles of medical documentation applicable to all medical services. The bulk of the guidelines provide the rules for selecting a level of E/M service. The 1995 and 1997 guidelines are currently in effect, and clinicians are permitted to use whichever set is more beneficial to them in documenting a service and selecting the level of service. The key components of E/M services are history, exam, and medical decision making.

Clinicians generally prefer the 1995 guidelines, which have broader exam definitions. The 1997 guidelines allow clinicians to document the status of three chronic diseases as the history of the present illness (instead of the elements of the HPI), and had a much more specific multi-system exam. Auditors like this exam because it is less ambiguous than the 1995 exam. The 1997 guidelines also define a number of single specialty exams. These were especially helpful to psychiatry, ENT, and ophthalmology. Any clinician, not just specialists, may use these single organ system definitions.

Codes:

All codes are covered by the general principles of the documentation guidelines. E/M services are specifically defined by these guidelines.

Coverage:

Although these are Medicare implemented rules, they apply to all payers.

Billing and coding rules:

The Documentation Guidelines work together with the CPT® book to define the level of documentation that is required for each level of service for an E/M code. That is, they define what level of history, exam, and medical decision making are required for each level of service within each category.

The guidelines describe the documentation required for each of the four types of history: problem focused, expanded problem focused, detailed, and comprehensive. They define what is needed for each level of exam: problem focused, expanded problem focused, detailed, and comprehensive. In addition, the guidelines describe the criteria for the four levels of medical decision making: straightforward, low, moderate, and high.

However, to select a specific level of E/M code, providers and auditors must go back to the CPT® book, where the code descriptions include the level of history, exam, and medical decision making that are required. The CPT® book also tells you whether the code requires two or three of the three key components.

If time may be used as the determining factor to select the code, the times are listed in the CPT® book. There are some E/M codes for which time may not be used as the determining factor, including ED visits, and preventive medical services.

The following very important instruction can be found in the section of the guidelines called "General Principles of Medical Record Documentation":

> The CPT® and ICD-10-CM codes reported on the health insurance claim form or billing statement should be supported by the documentation in the medical record.

Coders and billers have taken this to mean that if it wasn't documented, it wasn't done. In a more complex way, this informs clinicians that what they tell an insurance company was done must be supported in the medical record. It sounds simple, but it is a very important principle. Whatever procedure and diagnosis codes are reported on the claim form must be supported in the medical record documentation for that date of service.

Related issues:

The Documentation Guidelines require that the legible identity of the provider should be noted in each entry into the medical record. The legible identity may be typed, dictated, or hand-written. However, if only the signature of the provider is in the chart, make sure you have a signature log which indicates that that signature belongs to a specific provider. Medicare does not require that office notes be signed. This differs from a hospital, where there are many regulations that require signatures in addition to the legible identity of the provider.

Key points:

- All entries into the medical record must be legible.
- The Documentation Guidelines provide the basis of the requirements for selecting a level of E/M service.
- The guidelines also describe general principles of medical record documentation that are applicable to all services.
- The AMA and CMS developed these guidelines jointly.
- Physicians and NPPs may use whichever set of guidelines is more beneficial to the provider.

See also: General principles of medical record documentation, time-based codes, E/M profiles, cloning notes

Citations:

CMS, *Documentation Guidelines for Evaluation & Management Services*, https://www.cms.gov/Research-Statistics-Data-and-Systems/Monitoring-Programs/Medicare-FFS-Compliance-Programs/CERT/index.html

CMS, *Medicare Claims Processing Manual*, Pub 100-04, Chapter 12, Section 30.6, http://www.cms.hhs.gov/Manuals/IOM/list.asp

Physician Auditing Workbook, Betsy Nicoletti, published by Greenbranch Publishing, www.greenbranch.com

Emergency Department Visits

Definition:

Emergency department visits are E/M services provided to patients in a facility that is open 24 hours a day for episodic non-scheduled care.

Explanation:

Emergency department services may be billed by physicians of any specialty, not just ED physicians. The physician does not need to be a regularly assigned physician in the ED to bill them. ED codes are only used in the Emergency Department, not in the office or outpatient setting.

Codes: 99281–99285

Coverage:

Most patients have coverage in their healthcare policies for emergency department visits. However, a payer may deny the service if the diagnosis that is submitted does not show that the patient needed emergency care. These are diagnosis-related denials.

Billing and coding rules:

Payers will typically pay for only a single Evaluation and Management (E/M) service per day per patient per physician. A physician who sees a patient in the emergency department, and later admits that patient to the hospital should bill for the initial hospital service only. The physician will not be paid for both an ED visit and a hospital admission on the same date. A physician may not be paid for an ED visit and critical care on the same date by Medicare. If a patient comes into the emergency room critically ill, bill only for the critical care time.

When a physician meets a patient in the ED to provide services on the weekend or after hours, and the location is selected for the convenience rather than for the necessity of ED services, bill outpatient codes 99201–99215.

According to the CPT® book, the amount of time spent with a patient does not affect the choice of the level of service for ED visits. That means that a physician may not use time as the determining factor in billing ED visits, and may not add prolonged services codes to the ED codes. However, a physician may bill for a procedure and an emergency department visit that are both medically necessary and are performed during the same visit. The E/M service—that is the ED visit—must meet the requirements of a distinct, separately identifiable service for a modifier 25 to be added.

Medicare pays physicians based on their group membership and on their specialty. So, it is possible for the ED physician, the patient's own physician, and a specialist to all be paid for medically necessary emergency department services performed on the same day.

Related issues:

Patients who are assigned to observation status and seen in the emergency department by a consultant should be billed using outpatient status as the place of service.

Key points:

- Any physician or NPP may bill for emergency department visits when providing services in the emergency department.
- If a patient is admitted to the hospital from the ED, bill only for the initial hospital visit. Payers will not pay for both critical care and ED care billed by the same physician on the same date for the same patient.
- If the patient's personal physician is called to the emergency department by the ED doctor to provide a service, bill for that using either the emergency department codes 99281–99285 or the outpatient and office visit codes 99201–99215. Do not bill a consultation for these services, because consultation was not requested.

See also: Consultations, hospital initial services, critical care.

Citation:

CMS, *Medicare Claims Processing Manual*, Pub 100–04, Chapter 12, Section 30.6.11, http://www.cms.gov/Manuals/IOM/list.asp

Evaluation and Management Services and Profiles

Definition:

Evaluation and Management (E/M) services are office visits, consults, hospital services, nursing home services, home services and preventive medicine services described in the first section of the CPT® book. The E/M profiles are normative data for the distribution of levels of service within each category of E/M code by specialty; they are commonly referred to as "bell curves."

Explanation:

E/M services account for a large percentage of all services billed by physicians of many specialties. Most of these codes are broken down into three to five levels of service, with varying documentation requirements for the history, exam, and medical decision making required to meet the criteria for that level of service. Some also have typical time assigned. Physicians and qualified NPPs may use either the 1995 or the 1997 Documentation Guidelines select codes for these E/M services.

CMS publishes annual data describing the distribution of each level of service within each category of service, by specialty. Medicare contractors use these data to compare individual physician profiles to the norm, and physicians and NPPs run the risk of audit if their profile differs significantly from the norm for their specialty. NPPs are compared with nurse practitioners and physician assistants rather than by the specialty in which they work.

Codes: 99201–99350.

Coverage: All payers.

Billing and coding rules:

The requirements for billing E/M codes are based on two resources: the CPT® book and the Documentation Guidelines. Each code listed in the CPT® book describes the level of history, exam and medical decision making that is required for it, as well as whether two or three of the three key components are needed. The descriptions, however are defined by the Documentation Guidelines and not explained in the CPT® book.

Developed jointly by the AMA and CMS, CMS posts the Documentation Guidelines on its web site. Currently, providers may use whichever set of guidelines is more beneficial to them, the 1995 or the 1997 guidelines. The 1997 guidelines included single specialty exams that were more clinically appropriate for some specialists than the general multi-system exam. The good thing about these guidelines is that they have been around for so long that many clinicians understand them fairly well, and countless cheat sheets, tools, and templates are available to make documentation easier.

Contractors and third-party insurances monitor the distribution of each clinician's E/M services by specialty and compare that with CMS norms. They do this within each category of service, such as established office visits, consults, subsequent hospital visits, etc. CMS publishes the raw data about code distribution by specialty on their web site, and many third-party vendors package this and sell it in an easily usable format. If an insurer finds that a clinician's distribution of codes is significantly different than other providers of the same specialty, it is likely to trigger an audit of selected E/M codes.

Clinicians should not bill all of their services at one level in any one category. That is, do not bill all your admissions as level two admissions, all your subsequent hospital visits as level one visits, and all your consults as level four visits. CMS expects that the acuity of patients' presenting problems and the complexity of patients' conditions vary, so the level of service clinicians provide, document, and bill will also vary.

The CMS norms are not meant to be prescriptive. Physician practices will vary. But if a particular physician's profile differs significantly from the profiles of other physicians in the same specialty, it's prudent to ask why. Some physicians consistently bill codes at a low level out of confusion about the documentation guidelines and fear of an audit, while others routinely bill all high level services. Some clinicians bill all services within a category at the same level of visit. Any of these patterns increases the likelihood of audit.

The Office of Inspector General (OIG) has released multiple reports showing that the level of service reported by physicians has changed to more high level codes. They suggested that CMS review the billing for providers who bill more than 95% of their E/M service at the highest two levels.

Related issues:

In the introduction to E/M coding in the *Medicare Claims Processing Manual*, CMS says this about selecting a level of service:

> Medical necessity of a service is the overarching criterion for payment in addition to the individual requirements of a CPT® code. It would not be medically necessary or appropriate to bill a higher level of Evaluation and Management service when a lower level of service is warranted. The volume of documentation should not be the primary influence upon which

a specific level of service is billed. Documentation should support the level of service reported. The service should be documented during, or as soon as practicable after it is provided to maintain an accurate medical record.

Use of an Electronic Medical Record (EMR) or paper template often makes it easy to document a higher level of service. Keep in mind that the medical necessity for the level of service is the most important factor in code selection, not the volume of documentation. The ease of documenting higher levels of service with electronic tools does not justify billing high levels of service for problems with low or straightforward decision making.

Key points:

- Practices should compare each clinician's profile by specialty with the CMS norms once or twice a year.
- If a clinician has a significantly different distribution, take the time to find out why.
- Some physicians have practices that legitimately differ from the norm.
- Audit the clinician's E/M records for accuracy.
- Provide coding education and ongoing support.
- NPP data are collected by Medicare without regard to the specialty in which the NPP works. This makes comparisons more difficult because the work and profile of a PA providing primary care services is certain to be much different from a PA working in oncology. Therefore, it is harder for practices to make realistic comparisons.
- A slight change in profiles results in a significant difference in revenue per office visit. If a practice finds significant undercoding, and through audits and education can change a provider's billing pattern, they can see revenue increases.

See also: Documentation Guidelines, Cloning

Citations:

CMS, Evaluation and Management guidelines at http://www.cms.gov/Outreach-and-Education/Medicare-Learning-Network-MLN/MLNEdWebGuide/EMDOC.html

CMS, *Medicare Claims Processing Manual*, Pub. 100-04, Chapter 12, Section 30.6.1, http://www.cms.gov/Manuals/IOM/list.asp

OIG Report, "Coding trends of Medicare evaluation and management services" May 2012, OEI-04-10-00180

OIG Report, "Improper payments of evaluation and management services cost Medicare billions in 2012" May 2014, OEI-04-10-00181"

Foot Care: Routine

Definition:

Routine foot care is defined as cutting or removal of corns and calluses, trimming, cutting, clipping or debriding of nails and other hygienic and preventive maintenance care, such as cleaning and soaking the feet, the use of skin creams to maintain skin tone of either ambulatory or bedfast patients, and any other service performed in the absence of localized illness, injury, or symptoms involving the foot. This type of foot care is not covered by Medicare, except in certain conditions described below.

Explanation:

Medicare does not pay for any routine services. However, if a patient has certain severe metabolic, neurologic, and/or peripheral vascular diseases, routine foot care may be covered. Routine foot care may be covered when these conditions pose a hazard to the patient when performed by a non-professional.

Codes:

11055	Paring or cutting of benign hyperkeratotic lesion (eg, corn or callus); single lesion
11056	Paring or cutting of benign hyperkeratotic lesion (eg, corn or callus); 2 to 4 lesions
11057	Paring or cutting of benign hyperkeratotic lesion (eg, corn or callus); more than 4 lesions
11719	Trimming of nondystropic nails, any number
11720	Debridement of nail(s) by any method: one to five
11721	Debridement of nails(s) by any method: six or more
G0127	Trimming of dystrophic nails, any number

Coverage:

Medicare covers this care for patients with these severe conditions once every 60 days.

Billing and coding rules:

Most Medicare contractors have developed a Local Coverage Determination (LCD) that describes specific diagnosis codes and conditions that show the medical necessity for a health care professional to provide routine foot care. It is critical to check the LCD annually. These diagnosis codes include diabetes, arteriosclerosis obliterans, Berger's disease, and peripheral neuropathies involving the feet. Covered indications also include chronic thrombophlebitis, and peripheral neuropathies involving the feet associated with malnutrition and vitamin deficiency, carcinoma, drugs and toxins, multiple sclerosis, and uremia.

Other conditions may also show medical necessity; the medical group must check with their contractor's LCD. For the service to be covered, the patient must be under the care of a physician of medicine or osteopathy during the six-month period prior to the service. In the absence of a systemic condition, the following criteria must be met. In the case of ambulatory patients, there exists: clinical evidence of mycosis of the toenail and marked limitation of ambulation, pain and/or secondary infection resulting from the thickening and dystrophy of the infected toenail plate. In the case of non-ambulatory patients, for coverage, there must exist clinical evidence of mycosis of the toenail and the patient must suffer from pain and/or secondary infection resulting from the thickening, and dystrophy of the infected toenail plate. In addition, procedures for treating toenails are covered for onychogryphosis or onychausix if there is marked limitation of ambulation, pain and/or secondary infection.

One LCD also notes these requirements: "The following physical and clinical findings, which are indicative of severe peripheral involvement, must be documented and maintained in the patient record, in order for routine foot care services to be reimbursable.

Class A findings
Non-traumatic amputation of foot or integral skeletal portion thereof

Class B findings
- *Absent posterior tibial pulse*
- *Advanced trophic changes as evidenced by any three of the following:*
  - *hair growth (decrease or absence)*
  - *nail changes (thickening)*
  - *pigmentary changes (discoloration)*
  - *skin texture (thin, shiny)*
  - *skin color (rubor or redness)*
- *Absent dorsalis pedis pulse.*

Class C findings
- *Claudication*
- *Temperature changes (e.g., cold feet)*
- *Edema*
- *Paresthesias (abnormal spontaneous sensations in the feet*
- *Burning*

The presumption of coverage may be applied when the physician rendering the routine foot care has identified:
1. *A Class A finding*
2. *Two of the Class B findings; or*
3. *One Class B and two Class C findings."*

There are three modifiers appended to the procedure code that describe these class findings.

Q7: One Class A finding

Q8: Two Class B findings

Q9: One Class B and two Class C findings

The medical record should document relevant history and physical exam and be specific. Document underlying medical conditions. The physician should also document the class findings that show the medical necessity and are reported with the Q7, Q8, and Q9 modifiers.

Related issues:

Complete an Advance Beneficiary Notice if the patient does not meet the criteria for covered foot care.

Key points:

- Medicare contractors have LCDs for routine foot care. Review the covered indications before providing the service.
- Document the history, the physical exam, medical decision making, and the procedure.
- Document the class findings in the note that support the medical necessity of the service and the modifiers reported.
- For patients who request routine foot care but do not have a covered indication or who request the care more frequently than allowed, obtain an ABN.

See also: LCDs, Advance Beneficiary Notice (ABN)

Citations:

http://www.cms.gov/Outreach-and-Education/Medicare-Learning-Network-MLN/MLNProducts/downloads/MedicarePodiatryServicesSE_FactSheet.pdf

http://www.cms.gov/Outreach-and-Education/Medicare-Learning-Network-MLN/MLNMattersArticles/downloads/SE1113.pdf

Contribution to this chapter from:

Mary-Ellen Schimmoller
Executive Director, Independent Networking Group, Inc.
   and
Hal Ornstein, DPM, FASPS
Co-Author, *31 1/2 Essentials for Running Your Medical Practice*
Managing Partner, Affiliated Foot and Ankle Center, LLP
Chairman, American Academy of Podiatric Practice Management
Chairman, New Jersey Podiatric Physician and Surgeons Group, LLC

General Principles of Medical Record Documentation

Definition:

The first two pages of the Documentation Guidelines discuss general principles of documentation for all medical services.

Explanation:

These first pages explain the importance of documentation in the medical record. These principles relate to all medical and surgical services in all settings, not just E/M codes.

Codes: All codes are covered by these guidelines.

Coverage:

All payers follow the basic CPT® rules, ICD-10-CM rules, and the Documentation Guidelines in paying claims.

Billing and coding rules:

The Documentation Guidelines tell us that this documentation is important to ensure high quality care. The documentation for a medical service needs to be sufficient to be used by that provider, and by any other current or future providers who see the patient. It also allows for claims payments by accurately describing what was done at the medical encounter. Good documentation can be used for utilization review and quality control evaluation and for data collection that may be useful for research or education.

What do government and private payers want? Third-party payers want accurate reporting of the procedure and the diagnosis codes that reflect the service provided. They also want to see the medical necessity for providing the service. As we know, medical necessity is required for payment of any service by third-party payers.

When you look at the general principles of medical record documentation, one of the first requirements is that the record must be complete and legible. If only the physician and the practice staff can read the note, that is not considered a legible record. Other physicians and healthcare providers who would need to care for that patient should be able to be read it.

Related issues:

Medicare and most payers do not require a signature to pay for a claim, but they do require the legible identity of the provider to be included in the medical record. Practices governed by Joint Commission on Accreditation of Healthcare Organization (Joint Commission) or rural health rules will have signature requirements. If the signature isn't legible, print, stamp or type the physician's name. Medicare has recently begun counting illegible signatures as errors.

Key points:

- Each patient encounter should include the reason for the patient's visit, relevant history and exam, and prior findings and diagnostic results. Each encounter should include an assessment or clinical impression or diagnosis. If the diagnosis is unknown, the patient's symptoms or complaints are documented as the clinical impression.
- The plan of care should be clearly written.
- The date and legible identity of the clinician should be documented.
- If tests are ordered, either the reason for those tests should be documented, or the reason for the test should be easily inferable.

See also: Documentation Guidelines, Cloning

Citation:

CMS, Documentation Guidelines for Evaluation & Management Services, http://www.cms.gov/Outreach-and-Education/Medicare-Learning-Network-MLN/MLNEdWebGuide/EMDOC.html

Global Surgical Package

Definition:

The global surgical package describes a set of services included in the payment for the surgical procedure.

Explanation:

Beginning in 1992, the Centers for Medicare and Medicaid Services (CMS) developed a single payment for surgical procedures that included certain pre-operative care, intra-operative care and postoperative care. Prior to 1992, a surgeon could bill for all Evaluation and Management (E/M) services before the procedure, on the day of the procedure, and in the days following the procedure. In 1996, the concept of bundling of surgical procedures was introduced. Current Procedure Terminology (CPT®) has also adopted the concept of a global payment for procedures with a slightly different definition of postoperative care. In the CPT® book, in the introductory section to the surgery section, CPT® describes the global package as including "typical" follow-up care. That means, atypical or unusual post op care may be reported separately, that is, billed.

Codes:

Surgical services with an indicator in field 16 of the Medicare Physician Fee Schedule Database (MPFSDB) that indicated a global period of 000, 010, 090, XXX or ZZZ.

XXX—the global concept does not apply

ZZZ—add-on code to a surgical code

Coverage: Surgical services.

Billing and coding rules:

Medicare defines the package this way. "The global surgical package, also called global surgery, includes all necessary services normally furnished by a surgeon before, during, and after a procedure. Medicare payment for the surgical procedure includes the preoperative, intra-operative, and postoperative services routinely performed by the surgeon or by members of the same group with the same specialty. Physicians in the same group practice who are in the same specialty must bill and be paid as though they were a single physician."

The surgical global period (in the MPFSDB) indicates the number of follow-up days included in the payment for the procedure. The end of the postoperative period is defined by these global days. Some minor surgical procedures and endoscopies have zero follow-up days, and some minor surgical procedures have 10 global days. Major surgical procedures have a 90-day global period. The global period starts the day of a minor procedure or the day before a major procedure.

The *Medicare Claims Processing Manual* describes those services included in and excluded from the global package:

Services included in the global package are the following:

- Preoperative Visits—Preoperative visits after the decision is made to operate beginning with the day before the day of surgery for major procedures and the day of surgery for minor procedures;
- Intra-operative Services—Intra-operative services that are normally a usual and necessary part of a surgical procedure;
- Complications Following Surgery—All additional medical or surgical services required of the surgeon during the postoperative period of the surgery because of complications which do not require additional trips to the operating room;
- Postoperative Visits—Follow-up visits during the postoperative period of the surgery that are related to recovery from the surgery;
- Postsurgical Pain Management—By the surgeon;
- Supplies—Except for those identified as exclusions; and
- Miscellaneous Services—Items such as dressing changes; local incisional care; removal of operative pack; removal of cutaneous sutures and staples, lines, wires, tubes, drains, casts, and splints; insertion, irrigation and removal of urinary catheters, routine peripheral intravenous lines, nasogastric and rectal tubes; and changes and removal of tracheostomy tubes.

Medicare lists these services as excluded from the global package.

These services may be paid for separately:

- The initial consultation or evaluation of the problem by the surgeon to determine the need for surgery. Please note that this policy only applies to major surgical procedures. The initial evaluation is always included in the allowance for a minor surgical procedure;
- Services of other physicians except where the surgeon and the other physician(s) agree on the transfer of care. This agreement may be in the form of a letter or an annotation in the discharge summary, hospital record, or ASC record;
- Visits unrelated to the diagnosis for which the surgical procedure is performed, unless the visits occur due to complications of the surgery;

- Treatment for the underlying condition or an added course of treatment which is not part of normal recovery from surgery;
- Diagnostic tests and procedures, including diagnostic radiological procedures;
- Clearly distinct surgical procedures during the postoperative period which are not re-operations or treatment for complications. (A new postoperative period begins with the subsequent procedure.) This includes procedures done in two or more parts for which the decision to stage the procedure is made prospectively or at the time of the first procedure. Examples of this are procedures to diagnose and treat epilepsy (codes 61533, 61534-61536, 61539, 61541, and 61543) which may be performed in succession within 90 days of each other;
- Treatment for postoperative complications which requires a return trip to the operating room (OR). An OR for this purpose is defined as a place of service specifically equipped and staffed for the sole purpose of performing procedures. The term includes a cardiac catheterization suite, a laser suite, and an endoscopy suite. It does not include a patient's room, a minor treatment room, a recovery room, or an intensive care unit (unless the patient's condition was so critical there would be insufficient time for transportation to an OR);
- If a less extensive procedure fails, and a more extensive procedure is required, the second procedure is payable separately;
- For certain services performed in a physician's office, separate payment can no longer be made for a surgical tray (code A4550). This code is now a Status B and is no longer a separately payable service on or after January 1, 2002. However, splints and casting supplies are payable separately under the reasonable charge payment methodology;
- Immunosuppressive therapy for organ transplants; and
- Critical care services (codes 99291 and 99292) unrelated to the surgery where a seriously injured or burned patient is critically ill and requires constant attendance of the physician.

Preoperative services

Preoperative medically necessary evaluations are separately payable from the global package, and these are discussed in more detail in the preoperative entry in this book. Physicians who provide the entire global package, i.e., preoperative, intraoperative, and postoperative care, should use a surgical code without any modifier. Medicare pays for physicians in a group practice of the same specialty as if they were one physician.

If a surgeon sees a patient and schedules the patient for surgery in 35 days, can the surgeon bill for a preoperative history and physical? No. Although the hospital requires a history and physical, once the decision for surgery is made and the surgery is scheduled, do not bill subsequent E/M services.

E/M on the same day as a minor procedure:
A minor procedure is defined as a procedure with 0 or 10 global days. An E/M service may be billed on the same day of a minor procedure only if it is a separate, significantly identifiable service, meeting the criteria of modifier 25.

Initial evaluation prior to a major surgical procedure:
Physicians may be paid for the E/M service at which the decision to perform a major procedure was made. That is, a physician can bill for a consult, emergency department (ED) visit, office visit, hospital visit, or other E/M service, which results in the decision for surgery that day or the next day. Append modifier 57 on the E/M service that was a visit at which the decision for surgery was made, when the visit is done the day of or the day before the major procedure.

This occurs in one of two situations:

- In the first, a patient is seen in the surgical office and the decision for surgery is made. In this case, the initial evaluation is paid, and the patient is scheduled for surgery. No modifier is needed.
- In the second case, the patient is evaluated in the office or the ED and a decision is made for urgent or emergency surgery to be performed that same day or the next day. In that case, CPT® and Medicare state this E/M service is payable, no matter what category of code or location of the service, as long as modifier 57 is appended to the E/M service.

Sometimes, a patient receives part of the global service from one surgeon and part from another. This may occur when a patient needs emergency surgery when away from his or her home, but the postoperative care will be provided back in the patient's home city. In that case, bill the procedure with a modifier 54 for the surgical care only, and bill the same procedure code with a modifier 55 for the postoperative care. Both claims should use the same date of service and the same procedure code.

Surgical services during the post op period:
Surgical modifiers exist for use when a surgical service is required during the global post op period. These could be staged or related procedures, repeat procedures, or planned or unplanned trips to the OR. There are separate entries in the book to describe these.

Unrelated follow up in the post op period:

The surgeon may bill for an unrelated problem in the postoperative period if the patient presents for an unrelated problem. For example, an orthopedic surgeon who had operated on a patient's knee could see the patient during the global period for a shoulder problem. The surgeon would bill the E/M service with modifier 24 to indicate it was an unrelated problem in the global period.

The CPT® definition of the global package includes typical follow-up services. Complications of the global surgical period per CPT® rules may be billed with the modifier 24. Medicare only pays for complications of surgery if a return trip to the OR is required.

Related issues:

Indicators in the MPFSDB break out preoperative, intra-operative, and post-operative percentages for surgical package work. Other indicators also identify surgical add-on codes, codes that can be billed bilaterally, codes which can be billed with a surgical assist, and codes which can be billed with co-surgeons or team surgery. All surgical offices should print or purchase a copy of this fee schedule annually.

Key points:

- The global period for a minor surgery begins the day of the procedure.
- The global period for a major surgery starts the day before a major procedure.
- Modifier use is critical to correct and accurate payment and reimbursement for surgical services.
- Payers will pay for medically necessary preoperative visits performed by medical physicians.
- The visit at which the decision for surgery was made if it is completed the day of or the day before the major surgical procedure, is billed with modifier 57.
- Consult the MPFSDB for important surgical indicators.

See also: Modifier 24, modifier 25, modifier 57, modifier 58, modifier MPFSDB, pre-operative exams.

Citations:

CMS, *Medicare Claims Processing Manual, Pub 100-04, Chapter 12, Section 40,* http://www.cms.gov/Manuals/IOM/list.asp

https://www.cms.gov/Outreach-and-Education/Medicare-Learning-Network-MLN/MLNProducts/downloads/GlobalSurgery-ICN907166.pdf

Healthcare Common Procedure Coding System (HCPCS)

Definition:

HCPCS codes are standard code sets used by healthcare providers and health insurance payers to report and pay claims.

Explanation:

HCPCS stands for Healthcare Common Procedure Coding System. Level one HCPCS codes are CPT® codes developed, maintained, and copyrighted by the American Medical Association. The level two codes are developed and maintained by CMS to describe services not defined by CPT® codes.

Codes:

There are over 10,000 HCPCS codes; these are found in the CPT® and HCPCS books, both published annually.

Coverage:

All payers use these codes to process claims. Coverage for individual services described by these codes varies considerably by payer.

Billing and coding rules:

Both HCPCS level one and two codes provide a standard code set that describe medical services and procedures provided by physicians and other healthcare professionals. The AMA maintains level one CPT® codes and describes them in the CPT® book published annually, in their annual *CPT® Changes: An Insider's View,* and in the *CPT® Assistant*, a monthly newsletter.

Having a CPT® code associated with a service does not necessarily mean that that service is reimbursed by payers. CMS publishes an annual MPFSDB. In this database, CMS assigns both Relative Value Units (RVUs) and billing indicators for each CPT® code. A code may be described by CPT®, have a status indicator of B (for bundled) in the Medicare database, and zero RVUs assigned. This tells you that this code is never billable to or payable by Medicare. Many private payers follow the bundling and status indicators and RVUs provided by CMS.

HCPCS codes are five digit, alpha-numeric codes that describe ambulance services, medicines, durable medical equipment, and some services which Medicare covers and defines differently than CPT® CMS also uses HCPCS codes to differentiate between diagnostic and screening services or to provide a distinction in coverage services.

CMS and the American Hospital Association joined together to be a clearinghouse to answer HCPCS coding questions. They refer CPT® questions to the American Medical Association (AMA). In years past, there were level three codes, which were local codes used by state Medicaid programs. With the advent of HIPAA, these local codes are no longer in use.

Related issues:

Along with ICD-10-CM codes, HCPCS codes are the standard code sets used by healthcare providers and payers.

Key points:

- Buy up-to-date versions of both the CPT® and HCPCS books each year.
- For medications listed in the HCPCS book, be careful about units. Depending on the medication, a practice may give one, two, or many units as a single dose.
- Supplies are described by HCPCS codes. Many supplies used in a physician office are not separately payable, but are bundled into the payment for the office visit or procedure. Medicare claims for durable medical equipment are processed by Durable Medical Equipment Regional Carriers (DMERCs) contractors, not by Medicare Administrative Contractors.
- Check with your private payers to see if they recognize services described by HCPCS codes.

See also: The Medicare Physician Fee Schedule Database (MPFSDB).

Citation:

CMS, http://www.cms.gov/MedHCPCSGenInfo

Hierarchical Condition Categories (HCCs)

Definition:

HCCs is a risk adjustment model developed by Medicare to pay Medicare Advantage plans. It estimates the expected health care costs for individuals for the next 18 months.

Explanation:

In fee-for-service medicine, diagnosis coding establishes medical necessity, and may be the reason for a denial, particularly for diagnostic tests or procedures. Services with national or local coverage policies often have specific diagnosis codes that are required for payment. In risk-based contracts or shared savings programs, payers assess the acuity of a panel of patients, and use that acuity along with age/gender distribution, cost, quality and outcomes, to provide incentive payments or decrease payments at the end of a contract year.

Codes:

Selected International Classification of Diseases, 10th Edition (ICD-10) codes.

Coverage:

This is the system the Centers for Medicare and Medicaid Services (CMS) uses to adjust payments to Medicare Advantage plans. Some medical groups are part of shared savings programs with Medicare or have risk adjusted contracts with commercial payers. Some private payers use proprietary systems to estimate risk and future payments, and some use HCCs. Using this system in medical practice payment is part of moving from volume to value.

Billing and Coding Rules:

The risk for an individual is determined by two things: demographics and diagnoses. A 65-year-old living at home has a lower demographic risk score than an 80-year-old living in a long-term care facility, who is dually eligible for Medicare and Medicaid. Demographic factors included in HCC calculations are age/gender, living at home or in an institution, End-Stage Renal Disease (ESRD) patient, and dual eligibility for Medicare and Medicaid.

Diagnosis codes assigned on a claim form during a calendar (or contract) year reported on an inpatient claim, outpatient hospital claims, or physician and certain other health professionals' claims are counted in determining the total risk score. Not all ICD-10 codes have a risk adjustment assigned to them. Those that do are assigned to groups, and groups have a specific weight.

For Medicare patients to Medicare Advantage plans:

Patient demographics	+	HCC diagnosis codes	=	Risk adjustment factor × CMS capitation rate

Diagnosis codes	➡	Diagnosis Groups

Diagnosis groups	➡	Condition Categories, and assigned a risk adjustment factor (RAF)

- Related conditions are assigned in one category and only the most serious is counted.
- Conditions in the same group are counted once. For example, morbid obesity and body mass index (BMI) of 42 are in group 22. The risk score associated with these conditions will only be counted once in calculating the RAF. Clinicians shouldn't assign all diagnoses assessed at the time of the visit that require or affect patient care or treatment.
- A higher ranked condition causes lower ranked conditions in the same category to be ignored. (There are a few exceptions to this.)
- Unrelated conditions in different categories are both counted, and their effect is additive in assigning a score.

Clinicians should follow ICD-10 rules.
1. Use the ICD-10 Clinical Modification (ICD-10-CM) codes that describe the patient's diagnosis, symptom, complaint, condition, or problem.
2. Use the ICD-10-CM code that is chiefly responsible for the item or service provided.
3. Assign codes to the highest level of specificity.
4. Do not code suspected diagnoses in the outpatient setting. Code only the diagnosis symptom, complaint, condition, or problem reported. Medical records, not claim forms, should reflect that the services were provided for "rule out" purposes.
5. Code a chronic condition as often as applicable to the patient's treatment.
6. Code all documented conditions, which coexist at the time of the visit that require or affect patient care or treatment. (Do not code conditions which no longer exist.)

A clinician should document underlying medical problems that require or affect treatment even if it's not being treated the problem at this visit. For example, a surgeon sees patient with kidney disease, diabetes, and heart disease, sending the patient for preoperative clearance. The patient's underlying medical conditions affect the surgeon's treatment of the patient. The surgeon should report these underlying conditions that affect the patient's treatment.

Do not report problems listed in the problem list or past medical history, which are not treated or which do not affect patient care.

Related issues:

Individual medical practice claims continue to be paid based on the fee associated with the Current Procedural Terminology (CPT®) or Healthcare Common Procedural Coding System (HCPCS) code. Groups that are part of an accountable care organization or other Medicare shared savings program or that have risk-adjusted commercial contracts will see an adjustment in their fees at the end of the contract year, partially based on the acuity of their patient population.

Key points:

- Follow ICD-10 rules when submitting diagnosis codes on claim form.
- Document those conditions treated, assessed, managed, or reviewed and submit the diagnosis codes for those on a claim form.
- Document those conditions that affect the care of the patient, and submit those on the claim form.
- Do not submit diagnosis codes for conditions that no longer exist. Use "personal history of" codes, when accurate.

See also: Diagnosis coding, ICD-10-CM

Citation:

https://www.cms.gov/Medicare/Health-Plans/MedicareAdvtgSpecRateStats/Risk-Adjustors.html

Hospital Discharge Services

Definition:

The services physicians provide on the final day of an inpatient admission are discharge services. Only the admitting physician may be paid for the discharge service. Other physicians seeing the patient on the last day of a hospitalization use subsequent hospital visit codes.

Explanation:

The discharge physician can bill for services provided to hospital inpatients on the final day of their stay using two CPT® codes, 99238 or 99239. These are time-based codes and do not have specific requirements for history, exam, or medical decision making, as other E/M codes do. The physician must have a face-to-face service with the patient on the day of discharge to bill the discharge codes, but the physician is not required to examine the patient. These services can include any of the following: physically examining the patient, discussing the hospital stay and instructions for aftercare to the patient and/or caregivers, preparing discharge records or referral forms, and writing prescriptions.

Codes:

99238 Hospital discharge day management, 30 minutes or less
99239 Hospital discharge day management, more than 30 minutes

Coverage:

Most health insurance policies provide coverage for medically necessary hospital inpatient services.

Billing and coding rules:

Discharge visits require a face-to-face service with the patient. Only one physician may bill for discharge services. Other physicians or consultants who see the patient on the final day of a hospital stay should bill with subsequent hospital visit codes. If a physician sees the patient more than once on the day that the patient is discharged, only the discharge service is billable. Payers will not pay for both a subsequent hospital visit and a discharge visit on the same day, by the same physician or by physicians in a group of the same specialty.

The Internet Only Manual (IOM) in the Teaching Physician Rules section (100.1.4) also instructs physicians that to use time-based codes, time must be documented in the medical record for either level of discharge visit. In common practice, physicians rarely document time for the lower level discharge visit.

However, to bill 99239 the total time of the discharge must be documented in the medical record.

Related issues:

Physicians can bill for a discharge visit from a hospital and admission to a skilled nursing facility on the same calendar date. However, to bill for the admission to the skilled nursing facility, the physician must see the patient in the nursing home and document the level of service required for the admission. Do not rely on the same documentation for both hospital discharge and nursing facility admission. If both services are performed and documented, bill both. If only the discharge is performed and documented on that date, bill only for the discharge visit.

Key points:

- Document time in the discharge summary for code 99239.
- A physician must provide a face-to-face service on the date of discharge to bill for discharge services on that date.

See also: Hospital subsequent services, hospital initial services, inpatient, hospital observation services, time-based billing

Citation:

CMS, *Medicare Claims Processing Manual*, Pub. 100-04, Chapter 12, Section 100.1.4 and Chapter 12, Section 30.6.9.2, http://www.cms.gov/Manuals/IOM/list.asp

Hospital Initial Services, Inpatient

Definition:

Commonly called the admission, the initial hospital care codes describe the first face-to-face encounter a physician has with a patient during an inpatient stay. Neither the word "admission" nor the phrase "history and physical" are descriptors in the CPT® book for this service.

Explanation:

The initial hospital service documents the reason for the admission; the symptoms or indications that led up to the admission; the patient's past medical, family, and social history; the examination of the patient; and the physician's assessment and plan. These services are per day codes. There are three levels of initial hospital services. For Medicare patients, starting January 1, 2010, the admitting physician adds an AI modifier to the initial hospital service. Report the initial hospital service on the day of the face-to-face visit with the patient.

Codes: 99221–99223.

Coverage: Covered by most payers.

Billing and coding rules:

Physicians should bill for the initial hospital service for the calendar date on which they have the first face-to-face service with the patient, even if that does not correspond with the date of admission to the hospital. For example, a patient is admitted to the hospital at 11:00 pm from the emergency department on November 11. The admitting physician comes into the hospital but does not have a face-to-face service with the patient until the next calendar day, November 12 at 1 am. The physician should bill for the initial hospital service on November 12. If the physician performs a subsequent hospital visit later in the day on November 12, the subsequent hospital visit will not be paid. All of the inpatient visit codes are per day, not per visit, codes. If the physician must see the patient more than once on the calendar date of the initial hospital service, only the initial hospital service is payable unless the patient is critically ill. Neither Medicare nor private insurance companies pay for multiple visits, as the description of the codes in the CPT® book as "per day" codes precludes this.

Only one physician can be paid for the initial hospital service for an inpatient admission. However, after January 1, 2010, consulting physicians who see Medicare inpatients will use the initial hospital services codes for the first visit during that admission, rather than using consultation codes.

When patients are admitted to the hospital by the same physician in the course of an ED visit or office visit, the physician can only bill for the initial hospital service. Two E/M services are not paid to the same physician in one day. However, an ED physician can bill an ED visit on the same day that another physician bills for the initial hospital service.

In general, health plans pay for one E/M service per day, per physician in the same specialty of the same group. Two internal medicine doctors from the same group cannot both be paid for hospital services to a single patient on a particular day. However, an internal medicine doctor and a cardiologist can both be paid for providing medically necessary services on the same patient, even if they are in the same group.

What if a physician admits and discharges a patient from inpatient status on the same calendar date? A series of codes (99234–99236) describes this service, admission, and discharge to observation or inpatient status on the same calendar date. Although this is more typical if the patient status is observation, the codes can be used for patients in inpatient or observation status. The physician must see the patient twice, once for the admission and once for the discharge to report a code in the 99234–99236 series of codes.

Whether a physician can bill for critical care and an initial hospital service on the same day depends on the situation. In general, remember that Medicare does not pay twice for the same work. If a physician admits a patient in the morning who is not critically ill, and the patient becomes critically ill later in the day, requiring a transfer to the ICU, bill for the admission in the morning and the critical care in the afternoon. However, if the patient was critical at the time of admission, bill only for the critical care time. See the section on critical care for more detail.

Initial hospital services have typical times listed for them in the CPT® book. Bill these services based on the total time spent on the unit doing the admission, if more than 50% of the total time was spent in face-to-face with the patient in discussion or coordination of care done while on the unit.

Related issues:

Physicians should document initial hospital services carefully. Although the patient's condition may warrant a level two or level three initial service, the documentation often lacks a comprehensive history or a comprehensive exam. Level two or three admissions requires a comprehensive history: level four history of the present illness items,10–14 systems reviewed in the review of systems, and all three of past medical, family and social history. Many admissions lack a complete review of systems and family history, and thus audit at the lowest level of admission. Also, level two and level three admissions require a comprehensive exam. For many physicians, this is an eight-organ system exam as described in the 1995 set of guidelines.

Key points:

- A physician should bill for the admission on the calendar date of the first face-to-face service with the patient in the hospital.
- In addition to the chief complaint and HPI, document a complete review of systems, all of past medical, family and social history, and an eight-organ system exam for all admissions. Then select your level of service based on the medical decision making, that is, how sick the patient is upon admission.

See also: Hospital discharge services, hospital subsequent services, hospital observation services, critical care, time-based billing

Citations:

CMS, *Medicare Claims Processing Manual*, Pub. 100-04 Chapter 12, Section 30.6.9, http://www.cms.gov/Manuals/IOM/list.asp

CMS, http://www.cms.gov/Outreach-and-Education/Medicare-Learning-Network-MLN/MLNEdWebGuide/EMDOC.html

Hospital Observation Services

Definition:

These are services provided to patients who are designated as "observation status" at a hospital. Although only a physician may write an order for inpatient or observation admission, the facility often determines the status of the admission. The physician's category of code (inpatient or observation) must match the status reported by the facility. Use place of service outpatient for patients in observation status.

Explanation:

There are times when a physician wishes to observe a patient in the hospital and expects the patient to go home within a short period of time. Instead of admitting the patient to inpatient status, the physician admits the patient to observation status. The patient may physically be in the Emergency Department (ED), in a designated observation unit, or in a bed that is more typically used for inpatient status. The location of the patient does not determine the status; the status is designated by the physician at the time of the patient's admission. The facility may change the status of the patient based on facility rules.

Codes: 99218–99220, 99217, 99234–99236, 99224–99226

Coverage:

Third parties and Medicare typically pay for observation services. Whether hospitals can bill separately for an observation admission depends on the patient's diagnosis for Medicare. This means that the financial incentives for physicians differ from those for a hospital.

Billing and coding rules:

If a patient is admitted to observation status in the course of an office visit or ED visit, the admitting physician should bill only for the initial observation services, 99218–99220. The physician should note the date and time of the observation admission. All other physicians who see the patient while in observation status should bill using office/outpatient visit codes or outpatient consultation codes. For Medicare patients, consulting physicians should report office/outpatient codes, 99201–99215. For commercially insured patients, use outpatient consult codes 99241–99245. Observation services do have typical time associated with them in the CPT® book.

CPT® added subsequent observation visit codes 99224–99226. The admitting physician uses these subsequent observation codes for patients with all insurances. For Medicare patients, the consulting physician uses office/outpatient codes for follow-up visits.

Observation billing raises a number of "what if" questions. Here are some common examples of observation billing.

In this example, the patient remains in observation status for part of three calendar days. This is not typical but happens from time to time. Bill the first day using initial observation status codes; bill the second day with either subsequent observation visits or outpatient/office visit codes because the patient is not an inpatient. Bill the final day using the observation discharge code. This is a CMS, not a CPT® rule.

Example 1	Bill with these series of codes
Patient admitted to observation status (OBS), April 1, 9:30 pm	99218–99220
Patient remains in OBS status, April 2	99224–99226 or 99212–99215
Patient discharged, April 3	99217

In example two, the patient is admitted to observation status, but the physician changes the patient status to inpatient on the same calendar date. Bill only for the initial inpatient service, not for the initial observation service.

Example 2	Bill with these series of codes
Patient admitted to observation status, April 1, noon	
Patient changed to inpatient status, April 1, 5 pm	99221–99223

The CPT® definition of the next set of codes is for admission and discharge on the same calendar date in observation or inpatient status. They have higher RVUs than the other initial hospital service codes because the work for the discharge is included in them. To bill these codes, the patient must be admitted and discharged on the same calendar date. Medicare has an additional rule: the patient must be in observation status for over eight hours to use these codes. Also, the physician must see the patient twice and separately document the admission and discharge.

Example 3	Bill with these series of codes
Patient admitted to observation status, April 1, 8 am	
Patient discharged to home, April 1, 5 pm	99234–99236

Hospital and physician status billing:

The status of codes reported (i.e., billed) by the physician should match the status reported by the hospital. If the hospital changes the admission status from observation to inpatient status, the physician coding should match. Prior to submitting a claim, the biller in the physician office should check the facility status of the patient.

Related issues:

The Relative Value Units (RVUs) and payments for initial hospital services and observation services are almost the same. The documentation requirements for these initial observation services are identical to the documentation requirements for initial hospital services. Physicians should remember to document a complete review of systems and past medical, family and social history. Without all three elements of the patient's history, the initial observation service will audit at the lowest level. The place of service for observation service is 22, outpatient.

Key points:

- Select observation codes based on the status of the patient in the hospital.
- Note the time of the admission to observation status.
- If a patient remains in observation status on the second calendar date, the admitting physician uses subsequent observation codes.
- When the patient status is changed to inpatient status, bill subsequent hospital visits.
- If a patient status is changed from observation to inpatient on the same date that the patient was admitted to observation, bill only the inpatient initial service.
- For non-Medicare patients, bill consults based on the status of the patient. Bill outpatient consults for patients in observation status and bill inpatient consults for patients who are inpatients.

- Use the observation discharge code to report discharging a patient from observation services, but do not bill for the discharge from observation and the admission to inpatient status on the same day.

See also: Hospital subsequent services, hospital initial services, hospital discharge services, time-based billing

Citation:

CMS, *Medicare Claims Processing Manual*, Pub. 100-04, Chapter 12, Section 30.6.8, http://www.cms.gov/Manuals/IOM/list.asp

Hospital Subsequent Services

Definition:

Subsequent hospital services refer to care provided by the attending physician to a hospital inpatient. Consulting physicians providing care to an inpatient after an initial consultation also use the subsequent hospital services code.

Explanation:

Commonly referred to as "daily rounds," subsequent hospital services include all of the daily care provided by the attending physician, including medical record review, history taking and examination of the patient, review of diagnostic results from the previous day, record keeping, and development of the assessment and discharge plan. The service also includes discussions with the hospital staff, other physicians, the patient, and the patient's family. The definition of the visits is for care of the patient for per day, so only bill one subsequent hospital visit per day, no matter how many times the physician saw the patient that day.

Codes: 99231–99233.

Coverage:

Most health insurance policies provide coverage for medically necessary hospital inpatient services.

Billing and coding rules:

These are per day, not per visit codes, so bill only once for a patient's care on a single calendar date no matter how many times the physician saw the patient that day. What if the physician is called back to the hospital later in the day? A physician can add the documentation for two visits to determine the level of service, and if documented, bill a higher level. But only one visit is payable. Likewise, if the physician's partner is covering for the attending physician, and the two physicians are of the same specialty, only one visit is payable for that date.

Multiple physicians of different specialties can bill for medically necessary hospital visits. That is, an internist, a cardiologist and a renal specialist may all bill and be paid for subsequent hospital visits on the same date if they are providing medically necessary services. Although different diagnoses will decrease the likelihood of an initial denial and need for appeal, they are not required.

However, only one physician may bill a discharge visit; other physicians of different specialties who provide medically necessary hospital services on the day of discharge should bill a subsequent hospital visit. A physician cannot bill both a subsequent hospital service and a discharge visit on the same day.

Subsequent hospital visits have typical times associated with them in the CPT® book, so a clinician may use time to select a subsequent hospital visit if more than 50% of the unit visit is spent face-to-face with the patient in discussion/counseling with the patient.

Bill for the calendar date that the physician saw the patient for subsequent hospital visits. If the patient was admitted on January 1 at midnight, and the physician had a face-to-face service with the patient at 2:00 a.m. and performed the initial hospital service (commonly called the admission), the physician will not be paid for a subsequent hospital visit at 10:00 a.m. on the same calendar date. Only one E/M service is payable per date for physicians of the same specialty in the same group, and additional subsequent hospital visits will not be paid.

Related issues:

Medicare has a third-party contractor conduct reviews of paid claims—Comprehensive Error Rate Testing (CERT)—to see if payment made by carriers to physicians is accurate. CMS finds that the documentation needed to support the highest level of subsequent hospital visit is frequently missing when they review the record. Two of the three key components of history, exam, and medical decision making are required. The required history is four elements of the history of the present illness, with two to nine systems reviewed; the exam 12 elements examined, using the 1997 guidelines; and the medical decision making is high complexity.

Key points:

- Bill only one subsequent visit per calendar date.
- Be careful about handwriting, because the documentation must be legible for the visit to be payable.
- If using an Electronic Health Record (EHR), use caution in copying notes from the previous day. It can lead to medical errors and inaccuracies. Document the history, exam and medical decision making taken and done at this date.
- Document a history of the present illness by describing the patient's symptoms or illness during the past 24 hours. "Patient sitting in bed," does not qualify as a history.

See also: Hospital discharge services, hospital initial services, hospital observation services, critical care, time-based billing

Citation:

CMS, *Medicare Claims Processing Manual,* Pub. 100-04, Chapter 12, Section 30.6.9, http://www.cms.gov/Manuals/IOM/list.asp

ICD-10-CM

Definition:

The International Classification of Diseases, 10th edition, Clinical Modification (ICD-10-CM) version is a medical diagnosis system adopted from the World Health Organization (WHO) code set. Hospitals, but not physicians, use the International Classification of Diseases, 10th edition, Procedure Classification System (ICD-10-PCS).

Explanation:

Claims submitted to third parties contain procedure and diagnosis codes that describe the medical services performed and the reason for those services. ICD-10-CM was implemented on October 1, 2015, after multiple delays.

Codes:

Approximately 70,000 valid ICD-10-CM codes exist. Although the WHO version contains 16,000 codes, the clinical modification version is larger and has been adapted by the Centers for Disease Control and Prevention (CDC) and the American Hospital Association (AHA) and used by the US healthcare system.

Coverage:

HIPAA covered entities must use ICD-10-CM codes.

Billing and coding rules:

The general guidelines for ICD-10-CM codes are extensive. Medical coders need to pay attention to the guidelines and understand how to use the index and to select codes from the tabular section. There is one section specifically related to physician/outpatient claims, and it is brief:

1. Use the ICD-10-CM codes that describe the patient's diagnosis, symptom, complaint, condition, or problem.
2. Use the ICD-10-CM code chiefly responsible for the item or service provided.
3. Assign codes to the highest level of specificity.
4. Do not code suspected diagnoses in the outpatient setting. Code only the diagnosis symptom, complaint, condition, or problem reported. Medical records, not claim forms, should reflect that the services were provided for "rule out" purposes.
5. Code a chronic condition as often as applicable to the patient's treatment.

6. Code all documented conditions, which coexist at the time of the visit that require or affect patient care or treatment. (Do not code conditions which no longer exist.)

Some unique features of ICD-10-CM include a 7th character extender for injuries and other adverse affects, a place holder code "x" for codes that require a 7th character extender but are not already six characters long and a greatly increased set of codes for pre-procedural and post-procedural complications of surgeries. Some of these complication codes are in the organ system chapter to which they relate, and some are in Chapter 21, injury, poisoning and certain other consequences of external causes. Predictably, with such an increase in the number of total codes, certain sections will be detailed. This includes Chapter 21 and external cause codes.

The transition from International Classification of Diseases, 9th edition, Clinical Modification (ICD-9-CM) to ICD-10-CM utilized mapping programs in electronic health records (EHRs). Unfortunately, this resulted in a problem lists with many unspecified codes.

Related issues:

The accuracy of diagnosis coding takes on added importance as practices move from fee-for-service contracts to value based contracts.

Key points:

- Diagnosis Coding establishes the medical necessity for services that were performed.
- Medical coders should pay attention to the general guidelines, with particular care paid to the guidelines related to physician services.

See also: Hierarchical Condition Categories, diagnosis coding

Citation:

https://www.cms.gov/Medicare/Coding/ICD10/

Immunization Administration for Vaccinations

Definition:

The CPT® book describes codes for the administration of vaccinations. CMS defines additional codes for administration of immunizations that are covered by Medicare as preventive medicine services.

Explanation:

Vaccine administration is separately payable from the vaccine serum itself. For some patients and some vaccines, states provide the vaccine to the medical practice free of charge. However, states have developed guidelines with age and frequency limits for the free provision of vaccinations. Some vaccines are never provided by the state, such as those related to travel to a foreign country. When a practice receives the vaccine at no charge, it bills for only the vaccine administration. The practice bills for the vaccine administration and for the vaccine itself if it has paid for the vaccine.

These charges are in addition to the preventive medicine services, which are billed separately. There are CPT® codes that describe this service, including base and add-on codes.

Codes:

90460 through 90474. CMS also developed HCPCS codes for administration of covered preventive medicine services. These are G0008 for the influenza administration, G0009 for pneumococcal administration, and G0010 for hepatitis B administration. CMS publishes an annual immunization reference guide. Download it every year.

Coverage: Varies, and can be diagnoses dependent.

Billing and coding rules:

Bill for the vaccine administration when the office administers the vaccine. Bill for the vaccination toxoid if the practice paid for the product.

The codes 90460 and 90461 are used to bill for the administration of a vaccine to patients through 18 years of age, with physician or NPP counseling. Code 90460 is for the first component, via any route of administration, when the provider who administers the vaccine also counsels the patient. Nursing or staff counseling is not sufficient to bill this code. Code 90461 is for each additional component provided on the same day, by the same means. This is an add-on code and would never be billed separately from the base code 90460.

Codes 90471 and 90472 are for the administration of vaccines including percutaneous, intradermal, subcutaneous, or intramuscular. Use 90471 to report the first component and 90472 for additional components.

Codes 90473 and 90474 are used for vaccine administration by oral or intranasal route. 90473 is for the first component and 90474 is an add on code for additional components.

Related issue:

CMS has developed HCPCS codes for administration of covered preventive vaccinations. These are typically diagnosis specific.

Key points:
- Select vaccine administration based on the age of the patient, method of administration, and whether or not counseling is provided by the clinician.
- There are a series of add-on codes for additional components. Add-on codes can never be billed alone; they must always be billed with the base code. They are defined as each additional component, so bill these codes with a number of units.
- For Medicare preventive medicine services, bill the appropriate HCPCS codes and related covered diagnoses.
- Do not report a nurse visit for a patient who presents for the administration of a vaccine. Report the correct administration code.

See also: Preventive medicine, preventive medicine services for Medicare patients.

Citations:

CDC, http://www.cdc.gov/vaccines/schedules/index.html

http://www.cms.gov/Outreach-and-Education/Medicare-Learning-Network-MLN/MLNProducts/downloads/qr_immun_bill.pdf

Incident to Services (Medicare)

Definition:

Medicare defines incident to services as services provided in a physician office to Medicare patients that are an integral part of and incident to a physician's treatment and plan of care.

Explanation:

Incident to services are provided in a physician office and billed as if they were personally performed by the physician. The claim is submitted using the physician's provider number and is paid at 100% of the physician fee schedule. There are two common services billed in the office as incident to. The first is a nurse visit, which may only be billed at the 99211 level. The second is for the services of a qualified NPP, and those may be billed at the level of services provided to an established patient. For the practice to bill a service as incident to, the physician must have seen the patient first for that problem and established a plan of care. NPPs must bill new patients under their own provider numbers. Only follow-up care that was initiated by a physician may be billed as incident to if the following criteria are met:

- The staff member providing the service is employed by the physician or the group that employs the physician. Leased and contracted employees are permitted.
- The physician who initiated the plan of care is in the office and immediately available to provide assistance. The physician's partner may serve this function in a group practice.
- The service being provided is follow-up care. Because the care is incident to, no new patients and no new problems on established patients may be billed this way.
- The service is provided in the office, not the hospital, outpatient department, or nursing home. It must be an expense to the physician.
- The physician that initiated the plan of treatment remains actively involved in the plan of care. The physician and NPP may alternate seeing the patient.

An NPP can see new patients and treat established patients for new problems, but the NPP must bill these services under his or her own provider number (not incident to the physician) and be paid at 85% of the physician fee schedule amount.

Codes:

E/M codes. A physician does not need to be in the office to bill flu shots, EKGs, lab services, or x-ray services because these are covered under a different statute and do not count as incident to services.

Coverage:

Incident to is a Medicare rule. State Medicaid programs often follow incident to rules. Check with other third-party payers about their rules for billing NPPs and nurse visits.

Billing and coding rules:

Incident to services are services or supplies furnished as an integral but incidental part of a physician's professional services. They must be the type typically provided in a physician office. They may not be reported to Part B on a professional claim in an outpatient department, Emergency Department (ED), inpatient unit or nursing facility.

These services must be performed under the direct supervision of the physician. That is, the physician must be in the suite of offices when the service is performed. The physician must have seen the patient for that problem first and establish a plan of care. The physician also must stay involved in the patient's care. Some practices alternate visits between a physician and NPP. If the physician is in the car, at the hospital or on vacation, bill the service the NPPs provider number. However, if another, supervising physician in a group practice is available and in the office, the practice may bill the service as incident to.

The employee providing the service must be an expense to the practice: an employee of the physician, an employee of the group that employs the physician, or a leased or contracted employee.

Incident to services provided in the patient's home are payable IF the physician and the employee are present when the services are provided. These situations are rare. For all practical purposes, incident to services are billed and payable in the physician office.

New patient visits may never be billed as incident to because they do not meet the definition of being part of the physician's plan of care. These services may be billed by NPPs under their own provider numbers.

Related issues:

Some practices bill all of their NPP services under their own provider number, losing the 15% reimbursement difference just for ease of billing and uncertainty about the rules. Practices that want to collect the revenue difference need to educate their NPPs about the rules for incident to services, and ask the NPP to indicate on the encounter form whether the service is an incident to service or a direct bill service. Because this is the source of so much confusion, educate the providers and staff annually about it. Incident to represents both a compliance risk and a potential revenue issue.

Key points:

- An incident to service is a service billed to Medicare as if the service was provided by the physician.
- Incident to services may be billed in the physician office but not in the hospital or nursing home for Medicare patients.
- Incident to services are paid at 100% of the fee schedule.
- The physician must initiate the care, stay actively involved, and be in the office immediately available when the service is provided.
- The staff member providing the service must be an expense to the practice.
- Do not bill new problems or new patients as incident to.

See also: Nurse visits, shared visits.

Citations:

CMS, *Medicare Benefit Policy Manual*, Pub 100-02, Chapter 15, Sections 60.1, 60.2, and 60.3, and CMS, *Medicare Claims Processing Manual*, Pub 100-04, 02, Chapter 12, Section 30.6.4, http://www.cms.gov/Manuals/IOM/list.asp.

https://www.cms.gov/Outreach-and-Education/Medicare-Learning-Network-MLN/ MLNMattersArticles/downloads/SE0441.pdf

Local Coverage Determinations (LCDs)

Definition:

LCDs are Medicare contractor-specific rules developed in the absence of Medicare national coverage or coding policies, or as an adjunct to national coverage.

Explanation:

CMS developed National Coverage Determinations (NCDs), which define coverage policies for medical services. These NCDs define when Medicare will cover a service based on the patient's condition, symptoms, or diagnosis codes. NCDs apply to all carriers and localities throughout the country. In the absence of a national policy, local Medicare Administrative Contractors (MACs) may develop their own policies, provided they are in compliance with national coverage and coding rules.

Codes: As selected by the MAC.

Coverage:

These are Medicare policies. Many private insurance companies have their own policy determinations.

Billing and coding rules:

LCDs provide guidance to the physician practice about whether a service is considered reasonable and necessary for a patient's condition, and when and at what frequency the service will be covered. These LCDs must comply with national coverage and coding rules, and they are secondary to national policies.

CMS's web site includes a searchable database of LCDs.

Each LCD provides general information, the contractor name, the effective and revised dates, a description of the CMS national coverage policy, and the geographic locale to which the policy applies. LCDs also list the range of codes, a description of the service, indications and limitations of coverage and/or medical necessity, specific CPT® codes, ICD-10 codes, coding guidelines, documentation requirements, and utilization guidelines.

Related issues:

NCDs and LCDs address the issue of medical necessity. If a physician recommends a lab test or medical service to a patient who does not meet the criteria for the service based on the LCD or NCD, and the physician and patient wish to proceed, the physician should obtain an Advance Beneficiary

Notice (ABN) prior to proceeding. This allows the physician to hold the patient financially responsible for the service.

LCDs and NCDs provide the physician practice with specific guidance about whether a service is covered and payable. Physicians may disagree with the medical necessity as defined by the policy, but the policy is specific and gives them the billing guidance they need.

Key points:

- Physicians should check their contractor's web site for LCDs for services they provide.
- Review the covered indications for the service.
- Develop a procedure to inform patients prior to providing the service when the service is not covered for their condition.
- Execute an ABN properly.

See also: National Coverage Determinations, Advance Beneficiary Notice

Citations:

CMS, http://www.cms.gov/DeterminationProcess

CMS alphabetical NCD listing: http://www.cms.gov/mcd/index_list.asp?list_type=ncd

CMS, Medicare coverage searchable database: http://www.cms.gov/mcd/search.asp?

Locum Tenens Billing

Definition:

Medicare allows a physician to bill for services provided by a substitute physician under a locum tenens arrangement when the regular physician is away.

Explanation:

A physician who is absent from the practice due to illness, vacation, pregnancy, or continuing medical education may elect to hire a temporary physician on a per diem basis or a fee-for-time basis. This substitute arrangement, which may continue for a maximum of 60 continuous days, is paid by Medicare following the rules for locum tenens billing.

Codes:

Modifier Q6 is appended to the procedure code on the CMS 1500 form.

Coverage:

This is a Medicare rule. Check with your third-party payers before using a locum tenens arrangement for their patients.

Billing and coding rules:

Physicians who are away from their practices may bill for the services of a locum tenens physician using their own provider number. The regular physician must be unavailable to provide care, typically due to an extended illness or a vacation, and the Medicare beneficiary must seek medical care. The regular physician pays the locum tenens physician on a per diem or a fee-for-time basis. The maximum period for this coverage is 60 continuous days. Once the first coverage day has occurred, days in which the locum tenens physician doesn't provide any service count toward this time period. When the regular physician submits the claim, append modifier Q6 to the procedure code in item 24D of the CMS 1500. The regular physician is required to keep a record of the patients seen by the locum tenens physician and billed using the Q6 modifier.

Providers may not bill for an NPP using a locum tenens arrangement.

Related issues:

Postoperative care provided by a locum tenens physician as part of the global surgical period does not need to be identified on the claims form. A locum tenens physician may also be hired by a group practice to provide services when a physician has left the group. The group may bill for the locum tenens services for a maximum of 60 days using the provider number of the physician who has left the group.

Key points:

- The practice bills for the services of the locum tenens physician under the regular physician's provider number when the regular physician is unavailable and the Medicare patient seeks care.
- Pay the locum tenens physician on a per diem or fee-for-time basis.
- The maximum time period for this billing arrangement is 60 days. After that period, another locum may be used, but it cannot be the same physician for more than 60 days. If the arrangement is expected to last more than 60 days, enroll the physician in Medicare.
- Append a Q6 modifier to the procedure code when submitting the claim to Medicare.
- Keep a record of the patients seen by the locum tenens physician.

Citation:

CMS, *Medicare Claims Processing Manual*, Pub 100-04 Chapter 1, Section 30.2.11, http://www.cms.gov/Manuals/IOM/list.asp

Medical Necessity

Definition:

Medically necessary healthcare services are those services that would be provided by a prudent physician to evaluate, diagnose, or treat an illness, injury, disease, or symptoms. The definition of what is medically necessary can be straightforward or slippery, depending on one's perspective.

Explanation:

All claims for medical services to Medicare and other third-party payers must be medically necessary for the claim to be paid. Healthcare providers indicate medical necessity by the diagnosis code on a claim form.

Codes: All.

Coverage: All.

Billing and coding rules:

The Medicare web site glossary defines medical necessity for beneficiaries this way:

> Services or supplies that: are proper and needed for the diagnosis or treatment of your medical condition, are provided for the diagnosis, direct care, and treatment of your medical condition, meet the standards of good medical practice in the local area, and aren't mainly for the convenience of you or your doctor.

According to the ICD-10 CM book's introduction, establishing medical necessity is "the first step in third-party reimbursement." The diagnosis code submitted with the procedure communicates this medical necessity to the payer.

Medicare and local carriers establish coverage policies for medical services based on the patient's condition, symptoms, or diagnoses. These national and local coverage determinations describe a service and the covered indicators for that service. If a healthcare provider intends to perform one of these services on a Medicare patient who does not have a covered indication or diagnosis, the provider must inform the patient prior to the procedure that it may not or will not be covered. This process of informing the patient prior to providing the service is completed using an Advance Beneficiary Notice (ABN).

Related issues:

Medicare also raises the issue of medical necessity in documenting E/M services. The use of templates and electronic health records has increased the volume of medical record documentation for some E/M services. CMS says this about E/M documentation:

> Medical necessity of a service is the overarching criterion for payment in addition to the individual requirements of a CPT® code. It would not be medically necessary or appropriate to bill a higher level of Evaluation and Management service when a lower level of service is warranted. The volume of documentation should not be the primary influence upon which a specific level of service is billed. However—be careful! Medicare never defines medical necessity and level of service. Coders should be extremely cautious in determining that a certain level of history or exam is not medically necessary.

Key points:
- Follow diagnosis coding rules in the ICD-10 book when submitting claims.
- Medical necessity must be supported by the diagnosis code on the claim form and by the medical record.
- NCDs and LCDs are specific coverage policies for healthcare services. Look at private payers' policies.
- Use an ABN if you are providing a service to a patient who does not have a covered indication for that service.

See also: National Coverage Determinations, Local Coverage Determinations, Advance Beneficiary Notice, Cloning.

Citations:

Introduction to ICD-10-DM codes

CMS, *Medicare Claims Processing Manual*, Pub 100-04, Chapter 12, Section 30.6.1, http://www.cms.gov/Manuals/IOM/list.asp

Medicare Physician Fee Schedule Database (MPFSDB)

Definition:

The MPFSDB is a file published annually by CMS, which gives relative value units, as well as other payment status indicators, which direct Medicare Contractors in the payment of claims.

Explanation:

CMS updates the MPFSDB annually on its web site. The MPFSDB includes relative value units for each CPT® code, geographic adjustments, locality indicators, and explanatory material.

Codes: There are 10,000 CPT® and HCPCS codes included in this file.

Coverage:

Medicare develops information that is then used by its carriers, private payers and physician groups. However, other payers are not required to use the indicators or RVUs in the fee schedule.

Billing and coding rules:

The fee schedule formula determines the payment amount for each covered physician service paid by Part B Medicare. Lab fees are not included, but values for lab services can be found in Medicare's lab fee schedule. The formula for payment is:

Non-Facility Pricing Amount =
[(Work RVU * Work GPCI) +
(Non-Facility PE RVU * PE GPCI) +
(MP RVU * MP GPCI)] * Conversion Factor (CF)

Facility Pricing Amount =
[(Work RVU * Work GPCI) +
(Facility PE RVU * PE GPCI) +
(MP RVU * MP GPCI)] * CF

The total RVUs for a service is the sum of the work RVU, the malpractice expense (MP) RVU, and the practice expense (PE) RVU. Each of these three components is multiplied by the Geographic Practice Cost Indices (GPCIs) for the location. That means an appendectomy performed in San Francisco is paid at a different rate than an appendectomy performed in South Dakota. Adding in the locality differences (i.e., the multiplication of the GPCIs in the formula) provides for different payments based on costs for the malpractice and practice expense components. The work GPCI is currently set at one by Congress for most states. Some pioneer states and Alaska have a higher work GPCI. If the GPCI for your area is less than one, the payment will be less than the national payment amount. If higher than one, the payment will be more than the national payment amount. When negotiating with commercial payers, it is important to know if the contract is based on local or national values, and which will be more beneficial to the practice.

There are two rates: non-facility (i.e., office or home) and facility (e.g., hospital, Ambulatory Surgical Centers, nursing facilities). The same service is paid at a higher rate in a non-facility (i.e., office) than in a facility.

The indicators in this file include a status indicator for each CPT® code; RVUs; global surgery days; surgical code breakdown of pre-surgery, inter-operative work, and post op care; multiple procedure indicator; a bilateral procedure indicator; and an assistant in surgery indicator. The fee schedule also indicates for each relevant procedure code whether co-surgeons or team surgery are payable and those codes covered by the endoscopy payment rules. The level of physician supervision of diagnostic procedures is indicated for diagnostic services.

Related issues:

The MPFSDB answers many questions for physician practices and provides much more information than relative value units.

Key points:

- Download the MPFSDB annually.
- Review the word file that explains the indicators for each CPT® code.

Citations:

CMS, *Medicare Claims Processing Manual*, Pub 100-04, Chapter 12, Section 20, http://www.cms.gov/Manuals/IOM/list.asp

https://cms.gov/Medicare/Medicare-Fee-For-Service-Payment/PhysicianFeeSched/

Mini Mental Status Exam

Definition:

The mini mental status exam (MMSE) tests cognitive function. One well-known example of this test is Folstein's Mini Mental State Exam.

Explanation:

Physicians or NPPs perform a standardized assessment to evaluate their patients' cognitive function. A number of these tests are available. They are typically performed as part of an E/M service.

Code:

There are no codes for mini mental status exam. When performed, the exam is part of an E/M service.

Coverage: As part of an E/M service, it is covered.

Billing and coding rules:

Physicians often want to charge for this assessment as a separate charge item. However, there is no CPT® code for performing a mini mental status exam. In the CPT® book, in the section on central nervous system assessments/test (e.g. neuro-cognitive mental status and speech testing) the CPT® book states: "for mini mental status examination performed by a physician, see evaluation and management code."

A series of codes, 96110–96120, describe psychological tests. It would be incorrect to bill for an MMSE using these any of these codes, however.

Related issues:

The 1997 documentation guidelines include a single specialty psychiatry exam. Clinicians who perform the components of the MMSE may find that using the 1997 guidelines, and the single specialty psychiatry exam in particular, they can more accurately document and bill for the service.

Key points:

- There is no separate billing for an MMSE.
- Bill for this service as part of your Evaluation and Management service. Examination is one key component when selecting a level of service for an E/M code.
- Look at the single specialty psychiatry exam in the 1997 guidelines.

Citation:

Mini Mental State Examination, http://www.minimental.com.

Modifier 22—Increased Procedural Service

Definition:

Modifier 22 indicates that a service provided was greater than is usual for that CPT® code. It is used on procedure codes, diagnostic tests, and procedures in the medicine section, but not E/M services.

Explanation:

Sometimes a physician may wish to indicate that the amount of work for the procedure performed was significantly greater than is typical. This could be because of extensive trauma, patient complications, unusual anatomy, or patient physical status factors. The CMS manual says this about modifiers for unusual services:

> The fees for services represent the average work effort and practice expenses required to provide a service. For any given procedure code, there could typically be a range of work effort or practice expense required to provide the service. Thus, carriers may increase or decrease the payment for a service only under very unusual circumstances based upon review of medical records and other documentation.

The CPT® book defines modifier 22 as "Increased Procedural Services: When the work required to provide a service is substantially greater than typically required to provide a service is substantially greater than typically required, it may be identified by adding modifier 22 to the usual procedure code. Documentation must support the substantial additional work and the reason for the additional work (ie, increased intensity, time, technical difficulty of procedure, severity of patient's condition, physical and mental effort required). Note: This modifier should not be appended to an E/M service."

> Chapter 1 of the NCCI manual adds this information:

> By definition, this modifier would be used in *unusual* circumstances; routine use of the modifier is inappropriate as this practice would suggest cases routinely have unusual circumstances. When an unusual or extensive service is provided, it is more appropriate to utilize modifier 22 than to report a separate code that does not accurately describe the service provided.

Use modifier 22 only for those services that represent significantly more work than is typical. As a rule of thumb, the additional work performed should be 25% more than normal.

Codes:

Use modifier 22 on anesthesia, surgery, radiology, laboratory, and pathology codes and on procedures in the medicine section.

Coverage:

Medicare and most third-party payers recognize the 22 modifier and pay additional reimbursement for its use.

Billing and coding rules:

Append this modifier to the procedure code. The payer will require additional documentation that demonstrates the significant extra work in the procedure report. A brief cover letter that supports and outlines the increased work is usually helpful. Have this additional documentation ready when the claim is electronically submitted, so when the payer asks for the additional documentation, it can be sent immediately.

If additional diagnoses support the additional work performed, be sure to document them in the medical record and include them on the claim form.

Increase your fee for this service before you send in the claim.

Related issue:

Do not use modifier 22 on Evaluation and Management codes. Be sure that the diagnosis coding supports the increased work.

Key points:

- Append when the increased work is significantly more than is typical for that procedure.
- The documentation should clearly indicate the additional work.
- Send a cover letter that briefly outlines the additional work and will support your claim.
- Use this modifier sparingly in those cases that are outliers.

See also: Modifier 52.

Citation:

CMS, *Medicare Claims Processing Manual*, Pub 100-04, Chapter 12, Section 20.4.6, http://www.cms.gov/Manuals/IOM/list.asp

Modifier 24—Unrelated E/M Service During a Postoperative Period

Definition:

Modifier 24 appended to an Evaluation and Management (E/M) service indicates that an unrelated E/M service was provided by the same physician during a global postoperative period.

Explanation:

The global payment for a surgical procedure includes the preoperative work the day of or the day before surgery, the procedure, and the follow-up for 0, 10, or 90 days. If the surgeon sees a patient during the global period for a problem unrelated to the surgery, appending modifier 24 to the E/M service allows the claim to be paid per CPT® rules. This indicates that this service was unrelated to the normal global postoperative care. Current Procedural Terminology (CPT®) describes modifier 24 as Unrelated Evaluation and Management Service by the Same Physician or Other Qualified Health Care Professional During a Postoperative Period: The physician may need to indicate that an Evaluation and Management service was performed during a postoperative period for a reason(s) unrelated to the original procedure. This circumstance may be reported by adding modifier 24 to the appropriate level of E/M service.

Codes: This modifier is appended to E/M services.

Coverage:

Most payers recognize modifier 24. However, Centers for Medicare and Medicaid Services (CMS) defines follow-up during the postoperative period differently than CPT®. Medicare, per CMS rules, will only pay for complications of surgery if a return trip to the Operating Room (OR) is required. The CPT® definition allows payment of E/M services during the postoperative period for complications of the surgery, such as infection or wound dehiscence. A practice may report an atypical follow-up E/M service to a commercial payer, per CPT® rules. Modifier 24 does not perfectly describe that situation but is the modifier many payers require in this situation. This is an instance in which the Medicare rules and CPT® rules differ.

Billing and coding rules:

CPT® codes for surgical procedures are assigned global days (0, 10, or 90 days) in the Medicare Physician Fee Schedule Database (MPFSDB). Payment for normal postoperative care of the patient by that surgeon or by another surgeon of the same group in the same specialty is included in the fee for that surgery. However, if the patient is seen for an unrelated problem this service can be billed using a modifier 24. Non-Medicare payers that follow the CPT® postoperative rules may also accept this modifier on E/M services in the postoperative period for atypical follow-up.

Here's an example: An orthopedic surgeon sees a patient for follow-up from a knee arthroscopy. The patient, however, returns to the surgeon during that postoperative period with a wrist pain and numbness and is diagnosed with carpal tunnel syndrome. That surgeon may bill for an E/M service during the global period by indicating that the carpal tunnel syndrome was not related to the surgery. This is done in two ways on the claim form: append modifier 24 to the E/M code, and use a different diagnosis code than the knee problem.

Related issues:

CMS posts the MPFSDB on its web site annually. This fee schedule is the source of significant, important data for physician practices, including the number of postoperative days for each surgical procedure. It can be downloaded in an Excel file.

The definition of the global surgical package continues to vary between CMS and the AMA as defined in the CPT® book. This difference requires practices to have separate billing policies depending on the patient's insurance. If possible, when negotiating with third-party payers, add in a clause that states that the payer will follow CPT® postoperative rules. Check with private payers about the use of modifier 24 in this situation.

Key points:
- Different diagnosis codes are critical when billing with modifier 24.
- If both problems are addressed at the visit, document the new problem carefully.

See also: Global surgical period, Medicare Physician Fee Schedule Database

Citations:

https://cms.gov/Medicare/Medicare-Fee-For-Service-Payment/PhysicianFeeSched/

CMS, *Medicare Claims Processing Manual*, Pub 100-04, Chapter 12, Sections 30.6.6, 30.6.8, 30.6.9, 30.6.12, 40

http://www.cms.gov/manuals/IOM/list.asp

Modifier 25—Significant, Separately Identifiable E/M Service on the Same Day of the Procedure or Other Service

Definition:

Modifier 25 indicates that a significant, separately identifiable Evaluation and Management service was provided on the same day as a surgical procedure with 0 or 10 global days.

The CPT® book defines modifier 25 as follows:

Significant, Separately Identifiable Evaluation and Management Service by the Same Physician or Other Qualified Health Care Professional on the Same Day of the Procedure or Other Service: It may be necessary to indicate that on the day a procedure or service identified by a CPT® code was performed, the patient's condition required a significant, separately identifiable E/M service above and beyond the other service provided or beyond the usual preoperative and postoperative care associated with the procedure that was performed. A significant, separately identifiable E/M service is defined or substantiated by documentation that satisfies the relevant criteria for the respective E/M service to be reported (see Evaluation and Management Services Guidelines for instructions on determining level of E/M service). The E/M service may be prompted by the symptom or condition for which the procedure and/or service was provided. As such, different diagnoses are not required for reporting of the E/M services on the same date. This circumstance may be reported by adding modifier 25 to the appropriate level of E/M service. Note: This modifier is not used to report an E/M service that resulted in a decision to perform surgery. See modifier 57. For significant, separately identifiable non-E/M services, see modifier 59.

Explanation:

Payers will typically pay for only one service on a calendar date, either an E/M code or a surgery/procedure code. However, modifier 25 allows you to indicate to the payer that you performed a minor significant, separately identifiable E/M service on the same day as a procedure. Using modifier 25, a practice can be paid for an office visit—or any other E/M service—on the same day as a procedure that has 0 or 10 global days, if the E/M service is distinct. Modifier

25 is appended to the E/M service code, not to the procedure code. It is not needed for laboratory work or x-rays taken on the same day as the office visit according to CPT® rules, but some private payer editing systems require it for these services.

Modifier 25 is also used when billing an office visit (99201–99215) on the same day as a preventive medicine service to indicate that a significant, separately identifiable service was done on the same day.

Codes: Applicable to E/M codes.

Coverage: Most national payers recognize modifier 25.

Billing and coding rules:

When using modifier 25, the same diagnosis can be used for the E/M service and procedure. Typical pre-procedure work includes assessment of the surgical site, querying the patient about contraindications, and obtaining consent. The decision to perform the procedure is included in the payment for the procedure itself.

The National Correct Coding Initiative (NCCI) updated the chapter on reporting an E/M service with modifier 25. It states, "If a procedure has a global period of 000 or 010 days, it is defined as a minor surgical procedure. *E&M services on the same date of service as the minor surgical procedure are included in the payment for the procedure.* The decision to perform a minor surgical procedure is included in the payment for the minor surgical procedure and should not be reported separately as an E&M service. However, a significant and separately identifiable E&M service unrelated to the decision to perform the minor surgical procedure is separately reportable with modifier 25. The E&M service and minor surgical procedure do not require different diagnoses. If a minor surgical procedure is performed on a new patient, the same rules for reporting E&M services apply. The fact that the patient is "new" to the provider is not sufficient alone to justify reporting an E&M service on the same date of service as a minor surgical procedure."

Reading this definition carefully, it isn't always clear when an E/M service is separately reportable. An E/M service is separately reportable when the patient's condition must be evaluated prior to the decision to perform the procedure. A patient who presents with warts and says, "Can you freeze these off" should be billed only for the wart destruction. A patient who presents for evaluation of dysfunctional uterine bleeding and whose physician evaluates the symptom and decides to perform an endometrial biopsy in the course of the visit may be billed for both services.

A patient presents to an Orthopedic office for evaluation of knee pain. The Orthopedist takes a history, does an exam, hears about failed physical therapy treatment, and decides to do a joint injection. That day, report an E/M service, the medication, and the injection. The physician tells the patient to return the next two weeks for an additional injection. On the return visits, report only the injection and the medication.

Use this modifier on codes when the procedure has a 0 to 10 day global period. If the procedure has a global period of 90 days, do not use modifier 25.

The clinician should document that the service provided was separate from the surgical procedure. It is more likely to be billable the first time the provider sees a patient for a problem and must perform an assessment prior to doing the procedure. The E/M service is less likely to be a significant, separately identifiable service on visits scheduled for repeat surgical procedures.

For new patients, watch the level of exam that is documented. New patients and consults require all three components at the highest level. If the exam documentation is minimal on the day that the procedure is performed, make sure that the documentation requirements for that code are met. A low level E/M service is indicated in these circumstances. Payment for the decision to perform the procedure is included in the payment for the procedure itself.

Related issues:

In November 2005, the Office of Inspector General (OIG) reported on an investigation of claims filed with modifier 25, and reported a high error rate. According to the report, in 2002, CMS paid out $1.96 billion for claims that had a modifier 25 submitted. The OIG had certified professional coders review 450 of these claims, and 35% did not meet the program requirement for using modifier 25. In the sample, 35% should not have been billed as an office visit on the same day as the surgical procedure. They also found a large number of claims where modifier 25 was unnecessary.

The OIG recommended that CMS instruct its contractors about the use of modifier 25 and have the contractors work with physicians in learning the rules. The OIG also suggested that CMS should reinforce its requirements for billing an E/M provided on the same day as a surgical procedure. The service documented must entail significantly more pre-work and post-work than is typically associated with a surgical procedure. The OIG recommended that carriers emphasize the appropriate documentation of both the E/M service and the surgical procedure.

Key points:
- Append modifier 25 to the E/M code, not the surgical code.

- Use modifier 25 if the E/M service was a significant, separately identifiable service.
- Document both services carefully. Be sure that sufficient history, exam, and medical decision making are documented to justify and E/M service. Document the procedure fully.
- Use modifier 25 when the surgical service has 0 or 10 global days.
- For a scheduled procedure, report only the procedure.
- Different diagnosis codes are not required.

See also: Global surgical period

Citations:

CMS, National Correct Coding Initiatives overview,

https://www.cms.gov/Medicare/Coding/NationalCorrectCodInitEd/index.html

OIG, Use of Modifier 25, November 2005, Pub. OEI-07-03-00470, http://oig.hhs.gov/oei/reports/oei-07-03-00470.pdf

Modifier 26—Professional Component

Definition:

When only the professional component of a service is performed for a diagnostic procedure, append modifier 26 to the CPT® code.

Explanation:

Some diagnostic tests have both a technical and a professional component. These can be billed globally without a modifier to indicate that both components of the service were performed. However, in some instances, different physicians or a physician and a hospital may each provide one part of the service.

Codes:

Modifier 26 indicates that the professional component of a diagnostic procedure was provided, while modifier TC indicates that the technical component of a diagnostic service was performed. The CPT® definition is "Professional Component: Certain procedures are a combination of a physician component and a technical component. When the physician component is reported separately, the service may be identified by adding modifier 26 to the usual procedure number."

Coverage: Most third-party payers follow these guidelines.

Billing and coding rules:

Bill for the service performed—the technical component, the professional component, or globally—depending on what you have done in your office.

A common example is in radiology. A patient who receives a chest x-ray at the hospital will receive two bills for that service. The technical component of the chest x-ray will be billed by the hospital, and the professional component (reading the x-ray) will be billed by the radiologist who reads the film. However, if the physician provides this service in the office, owns the equipment, and interprets the x-ray, the physician will bill globally for the service.

The technical component of a diagnostic test includes providing the equipment, the supplies to run the equipment, and paying the staff to perform the test. The professional component includes the professional interpretation of the test.

The professional component is paid only once. An x-ray, which is read by an emergency department physician and then later read by a radiologist, can only be billed to the third-party payer once.

The documentation for the professional component in a physician office should include "radiology-quality reports." It is insufficient to simply sign a machine-generated report. Include in your report the indication for the test, the description of the test, and the test results.

Related issue:

One of the indicators in the MPFSDB is an indicator that denotes that a diagnostic test has both a technical and a professional component. A practice can also determine if the service has both components by looking at its listing in the MPFSDB. Services that have both components are listed three times: once as the global service, once with the Relative Value Units (RVUs) for the technical component and once with the RVUs for the professional component.

Key points:

- Bill for the service provided: the professional component with a 26 modifier, the technical component with a TC modifier, or globally without a modifier if both were provided by the same group.
- The total payment is the same, whether the service is billed globally or by its component parts.
- To bill for the technical component, the practice must bear the expense for the service. This includes owning or leasing the equipment, paying the rent, paying for the supplies to perform the test, and paying for the staff to do the test.

See also: Medicare Physician Fee Schedule Database

Citations:

CMS, https://www.cms.gov/Medicare/Coding/NationalCorrectCodInitEd/index.html

CMS, https://cms.gov/Medicare/Medicare-Fee-For-Service-Payment/PhysicianFeeSched/

Modifier 33—Preventive Service

Definition:

Modifier 33 is appended to a Healthcare Common Procedure Coding System (HCPCS) or CPT® code to indicate that the service is a preventive service, meeting the US Preventive Services Task Force Guidelines (USPSTF). This modifier was new in 2011. When the primary purpose of the service is the delivery of an evidence-based service in accordance with a US Preventive Services Task Force A or B rating in effect and other preventive services identified in preventive services mandates (legislative or regulatory), the service may be identified by appending modifier 33, Preventive Service, to the service. For separately reported services specifically identified as preventive, the modifier should not be used."

Explanation:

The Affordable Care Act mandated that services with an A or B rating from the USPSTF be covered by Medicare and group health plans without a patient due co-pay or deductible. A medical group or healthcare provider can indicate this by appending modifier 33 to the service. CMS also developed modifier PT, used when a screening colonoscopy is converted to a diagnostic or therapeutic service.

Codes:

CPT® and HCPCS codes that describe preventive services given an A or B rating by the USPSTF.

Coverage:

Medicare and private, group health insurances.

Billing and coding rules:

Append this modifier to the CPT® or HCPCS codes that describe preventive care services that have an A or B rating from the USPSTF. Although it is not required by many payers, it tells the payer that the service was a preventive service. Many commercial payers (and Medicare) pay for these services with an A or B rating without any patient due co-pay or deductible amount. Not all services are covered for both genders and at all ages.

Related issues:

See also modifier PT for colonoscopy services.

Key points:
- Check the USPSTF web site for an up-to-date listing of services with an A or B rating.
- Append modifier 33 to the CPT® code.

See also: Preventive medicine services. Wellness Visits, Modifier PT.

Citation:

CPT® Assistant, American Medical Association, December 2010/Volume 20, Issue 12, pages 3-6.

Modifier 50—Bilateral Procedure

Definition:

Modifier 50 is appended to surgical procedures and diagnostic services to indicate that a bilateral service was provided on the same patient, by the same provider, during the same session, and the service is not already defined as a bilateral service either by CPT® or in the Medicare fee schedule.

Explanation:

If a bilateral procedure is performed by a physician in one session, the surgeon may indicate that the procedure was bilateral by appending modifier 50 to the CPT® code selected.

Codes:

Modifier 50 is valid on the CPT® codes indicated as status "1" in the MPFSDB in the bilateral indicator field. It may also be used on radiology codes performed bilaterally.

Coverage:

Medicare pays 150% of the global amount of a unilateral procedure for bilateral procedures.

Billing and coding rules:

CPT® defines modifier 50 as "Bilateral Procedure: Unless otherwise identified in the listings, bilateral procedures that are performed at the same session, should be identified by adding modifier 50 to the appropriate 5 digit code." Some payers prefer that the claims for bilateral procedures be submitted to them on a single line on the insurance form with one unit and a 50 modifier appending the procedure code. Some other payers, however, prefer to have the claim submitted on two lines. The first line will indicate one unit with that procedure code, while the second line will indicate one unit with the procedure code and a 50 modifier appended. Practices need to check with each payer for instructions on submitting claims for bilateral procedures.

In general, using modifier 50 on a unilateral code will increase your payment to 150%. For x-rays, the payment is full fee for both services.

Read the CPT® definitions carefully, however, because you may not append a modifier 50 to a procedure code that is already defined as bilateral or as "unilateral or bilateral." Review the status indicators for bilateral codes in the Medicare database fee schedule.

Bilateral indicators, per the MFSDB:

0: 150% payment adjustment for bilateral procedures does not apply.

These codes are ineligible for the bilateral modifier because the anatomy or physiology of the human body is such that the procedure could not be done bilaterally or because the CPT® definition specifically describes the service as unilateral.

1: 150% payment adjustment for bilateral procedures apply.

A practice may append the modifier 50 to these surgical or x-ray services and be paid at 150% of the unilateral rate.

2: 150% payment adjustment does not apply.

The payment is already set at 150% because these codes are defined in CPT® as bilateral or the description says, one or both sides, or the procedure is typically performed bilaterally.

3: The usual payment adjustment for bilateral procedures does not apply.

These radiology procedures, when performed on both sides of the body, are not subject to the payment adjustment and will both be paid at full fee.

9: The concept does not apply.

Related issues:

The bilateral code indicator in the Medicare Database Fee Schedule tells physicians whether or not they can append a bilateral modifier to a code.

Key points:
- Check with third-party payers about how to submit claims for bilateral services.
- Do not use the bilateral modifier on any procedure that is described in the CPT® book or in the Medicare fee schedule as bilateral. Payment is already increased to 150% of the allowed amount.
- Do not use the bilateral indicators on services for which the MFSDB has indicated a 0, two, or nine indicator.
- Some carriers prefer a left and right modifier in place of the bilateral modifier, LT and RT.

See also: Multiple surgical procedures

Citation:

CMS, *Medicare Claims Processing Manual*, Pub 100-04, Chapter 12, Sections 40.6, 40.7, 40.8, http://www.cms.gov/Manuals/IOM/list.asp

Modifier 51—Multiple Procedures

Definition:

Modifier 51 is used when multiple surgical procedures are performed on the same day by the same surgeon, and the procedures are not bundled. Medicare contractors do not require it.

Explanation:

CPT® defines modifier 51 as "Multiple Procedures: When multiple procedures, other than E/M services, Physical Medicine and Rehabilitation services, or provision of supplies (eg, vaccines), are performed at the same session by the same individual, the primary procedure or service may be reported as listed. The additional procedure(s) or service(s) may be identified by appending modifier 51 to the additional procedure or service code(s). Note: This modifier should not be appended to designated add-on codes (see Appendix D)." This modifier is used for multiple surgical procedures performed on the same day by the same surgeon to indicate to the insurance company that a secondary procedure was performed and that the second procedure is not bundled into the first procedure. The first step is to determine which procedure is the primary procedure. The primary procedure is determined by looking at the relative value unit for each procedure, and is the procedure with the highest RVUs. Refer to CMS's MPFSDB for RVUs.

Codes: Append modifier 51 to the second surgical procedure.

Coverage:

CMS does not require this modifier when submitting claims. However, many private payers still use modifier 51.

Billing and coding rules:

When one provider performs multiple surgical procedures on the same day, bill by appending modifier 51 to the secondary procedure (when that procedure is not bundled into the primary procedure).

The primary procedure is paid at 100% of the fee schedule. The payment for the secondary procedure is subject to multiple payment rules. The surgeon is paid less for the second procedure. Medicare assumes that the physician will do the pre-procedure and post-procedure work for the primary procedure and does not need to be paid twice for the same work. Usually, the first procedure is paid at 100%, the second through fifth procedure is paid at 50% of the allowed amount.

Before submitting charges for multiple surgical procedures, always check the MPFSDB, as it determines which procedure has the higher RVU. Bill the procedure with the higher RVU as the primary procedure. Second, check the National Correct Coding Initiative (NCCI) edits. If the procedure is bundled and does not meet the criteria of a separate and distinct procedure, do not bill this second procedure. If the procedure is not bundled, bill it as the second procedure with a modifier 51.

There is a procedure in this book for determining whether to bill the secondary procedure and whether to use modifier 51 or 59 under the entry, "Multiple surgical procedures."

Related issues:

Some third-party payers use a claims-editing system that is not based on NCCI edits. This results in denials with a reason such as "this procedure is incidental to the primary procedure." Some practices successfully appeal these on a case-by-case basis by using the NCCI edits as a reference. Other practices have successfully negotiated contracts with third-party payers that require the payers to use the NCCI edits when processing claims.

Key points:

- When performing multiple surgical procedures, check the relative value units for each procedure. The procedure with the highest RVUs is the primary procedure.
- If the second procedure is a component of the first, and the second does not meet the criteria of "separate," do not bill the second procedure.

See also: Modifier 59, modifier 50, multiple surgical procedures

Citations:

https://www.cms.gov/Medicare/Coding/NationalCorrectCodInitEd/index.html

CMS, *Medicare Claims Processing Manual*, Pub 100-04, Chapter 12, Section 40.6, http://www.cms.gov/Manuals/IOM/list.asp

Modifier 52—Reduced Services

Definition:

Modifier 52 indicates to the payer the service was reduced. It means that significantly less work was done than would be typical for a particular procedure.

Explanation:

The CPT® definition of modifier 52 is Reduced Services: Under certain circumstances a service or procedure is partially reduced or eliminated at the discretion of the physician or Other Qualified Health Care Professional. Under these circumstances, the service provided can be identified by its usual procedure number and the addition of modifier 52, signifying that the service is reduced. This provides a means of reporting reduced services without disturbing the identification of the basic service.

This modifier is appended to a surgical service code to indicate that the amount of work performed for that service was less than typical.

Codes:

According to CPT® instructions, you can use modifier 52 when a service or procedure is reduced. However, CMS only recognizes modifier 52 when appended to surgical procedure codes.

Coverage: Recognized by many payers.

Billing and coding rules:

The definition for a surgical procedure describes all of the criteria that are required to bill for that service. If the physician performs only part of that service, however, and there is no other CPT® code, which more accurately describes the lesser amount of work done, append modifier 52 to the service. Use modifier 52 to indicate that part of the procedure was eliminated or reduced.

Related issue:

Do not use this modifier if the procedure was cancelled after the induction of anesthesia but before the service was commenced.

Key points:

- Practices will usually need to send notes along with the claim for this service.
- Do not use modifier 52 for discontinued services.

- The *Medicare Claims Processing Manual* specifically tells clinicians not to use this code for reduced E/M services.

See also: Modifier 22, Modifier 53

Citation:

CMS, *Medicare Claims Processing Manual*, Pub 100-04, Chapter 12, Section 30.6.1B, http://www.cms.gov/Manuals/IOM/list.asp

Modifier 53—Discontinued Procedure

Definition:

Modifier 53 is used for a discontinued procedure. According to the CPT® book, use it when the physician elects to terminate a surgical or diagnostic procedure due to circumstances that threaten the patient. Report the CPT® code of the discontinued procedure with modifier 53.

Explanation:

The CPT® definition of modifier 53 is "Discontinued Procedure: Under certain circumstances, the physician or Other Qualified Health Care Professional may elect to terminate a surgical or diagnostic procedure. Due to extenuating circumstances or those that threaten the well-being of the patient, it may be necessary to indicate that a surgical or diagnostic procedure was started but discontinued. This circumstance may be reported by adding modifier 53 to the code reported by the individual for the discontinued procedure." Modifier 53 is used on surgical or medical diagnostic procedures to indicate that the procedure was discontinued after anesthesia was administered to the patient due to a threat to the patient's well-being. It is not used to report a procedure, which was cancelled prior to anesthesia induction and/or surgical preparation in the operating room. Typically, the procedure will need to be re-scheduled because it was not completed.

Codes:

Use on surgical codes or diagnostic procedure codes. It cannot be used with E/M services.

Coverage:

Most payers recognize the modifier. The service is paid at a reduced rate.

Billing and coding rules:

The documentation should describe the clinical circumstances leading to the decision to stop the procedure. The note should indicate how much of the procedure was performed. Typically, the patient will be re-scheduled for the procedure. It is incorrect to use Modifier 53 when a procedure is converted from a laparoscopic procedure to an open procedure. In that case, bill only for the open procedure.

Related issues:

Not all modifiers affect payment, but all communicate to the payer that the circumstances related to the provision of service is different in some way.

Key points:

- Modifier 52 is used to describe reduced services. In that case, the procedure is completed, but not all components as described by the CPT® code were performed.
- Modifier 53 is used when the patient's well-being is threatened if the procedure is continued. The patient must have been prepped for the service in the operating suite and/or have anesthesia, and then the physician decided to stop the procedure.

See also: Modifier 22, Modifier 52

Citations:

CPT® Book, CPT® Assistant, Coding with Modifiers: A Guide to Correct CPT® and HCPCS Modifier Usage 5th Edition, by Deborah J Grider, published by the AMA

Modifier 58—Staged or Related Procedure

Definition:

Using modifier 58 on a procedure indicates that a staged or related procedure was performed by the same physician, subsequent to an initial service during the global period.

Explanation:

The CPT® explanation of modifier 58 is "Staged or Related Procedure or Service by the Same Physician or Other Qualified Health Care Professional During the Postoperative Period: It may be necessary to indicate that the performance of a procedure or service during the postoperative period was (a) planned or anticipated (staged); (b) more extensive than the original procedure; or (c) for therapy following a surgical procedure. This circumstance may be reported by adding modifier 58 to the staged or related procedure. Note: For treatment of a problem that requires a return to the operating or procedure room (eg, unanticipated clinical condition), see modifier 78." Use this modifier to report a staged procedure, which was planned at the time of the first procedure, or to indicate that the second procedure was more extensive than the first. It may also be used for a therapeutic service after a diagnostic one. Only use it during the surgical postoperative period for the first procedure.

The CMS manual has this additional explanation of using modifier 58:

Modifier "58" was established to facilitate billing of staged or related surgical procedures done during the postoperative period of the first procedure. This modifier is not used to report the treatment of a problem that requires a return to the operating room.

The physician may need to indicate that the performance of a procedure or service during the postoperative period was

a. planned prospectively or at the time of the original procedure;
b. more extensive than the original procedure; or
c. for therapy following a diagnostic surgical procedure.

These circumstances may be reported by adding modifier "58" to the staged procedure. A new postoperative period begins when the next procedure in the series is billed.

Codes:

Use on surgical codes. It cannot be used with E/M services.

Coverage:

Most payers recognize the modifier.

Billing and coding rules:

A physician may perform an abdominal surgery and plan to leave the wound open for a period of time. At the planned interval during the postoperative period, the surgeon takes the patient back to surgery to repair the surgical wound. Append modifier 58 to the second, planned surgery.

Related issues:

Physicians and coders must review the global days for the primary procedure to correctly assign modifiers during the global period. Physicians of the same specialty in the same group should bill as if they were one physician. That is, if a physician's partner does the second planned surgery, use the same modifier as if the first physician had performed the service.

Key points:

- Use modifier 58 on the subsequent service for a planned or staged procedure.
- A new postoperative period begins at the date of the second procedure.
- Do not use this modifier for complications of the first procedure that require a return trip to the operating room. Use modifier 78 for procedures performed as a result of complications.
- Use this when the second surgery is related to the first and is planned or staged.

See also: Modifier 78 and 79

Citation:

CMS, *Medicare Claims Processing Manual*, Pub 100-04, Chapter 12, Section 40.2, http://www.cms.gov/Manuals/IOM/list.asp

Modifier 59—Distinct Procedural Service

Definition:

Modifier 59 is a modifier of last resort, to be used only when no other modifiers accurately reflect the care provided. Chapter one of the National Correct Coding Initiative (NCCI) manual describes modifier 59 as follows:

> Modifier 59: Modifier 59 is an important NCCI-associated modifier that is often used incorrectly. For the NCCI, its primary purpose is to indicate that two or more procedures are performed at different anatomic sites or different patient encounters. It should only be used if no other modifier more appropriately describes the relationships of the two or more procedure codes.

CMS developed HCPCS modifiers to be used in place of modifier 59, but never implemented them.

Explanation:

The CPT® definition of modifier 59 is "Distinct Procedural Service: Under certain circumstances, it may be necessary to indicate that a procedure or service was distinct or independent from other non-E/M services performed on the same day. Modifier 59 is used to identify procedures or services, other than E/M services, that are not normally reported together but are appropriate under the circumstances. Documentation must support a different session, different procedure or surgery, different site or organ system, separate incision/excision, separate lesion, or separate injury (or area of injury in extensive injuries) not ordinarily encountered or performed on the same day by the same individual. However, when another already established modifier is appropriate it should be used rather than modifier 59. Only if no more descriptive modifier is available and the use of modifier 59 best explains the circumstances should modifier 59 be used. Note: Modifier 59 should not be appended to an E/M service. To report a separate and distinct E/M service with a non-E/M service performed on the same date, see modifier 25."

Modifier 59 bypasses NCCI bundling edits and allows a surgeon to bill for a secondary procedure that is bundled into the primary procedure. However, the secondary procedure must meet the criteria of being distinct and separate. This means that it is performed during a different session or encounter; on a different site or organ system; on a separate lesion, incision, or excision; or for a separate injury.

Codes: This modifier should be used on procedures, not on E/M services.

Coverage: All payers.

Billing and coding rules:

What constitutes a distinct and separate service? According to the NCCI, this could be a different session or patient encounter, a different site or organ system, a separate lesion, incision, or excision, or a separate injury. Different diagnosis codes are not required for Modifier 59 use. Use this modifier carefully.

NCCI gives coding pairs a Correct Coding Modifier Indicator (CCMI). If this is 0, then the two services may never be reported together and no modifier is allowed. A service with an indicator of 1 may be reported with modifier 59, if the definition is met.

According to CMS, modifier 59 may be used to bypass a bundling edit if:

There are different anatomic sites during the same procedure when the procedures are not ordinarily performed together

- At different encounters on the same day
- For timed procedures when the time periods are not contiguous
- For a diagnostic procedure that precedes a therapeutic procedure only when the diagnostic procedure is the basis for performing the therapeutic procedure

Related issues:

The OIG issued a report on the use of Modifier 59 in November 2005. It found widespread error in the use and payment of this modifier. Do not apply modifier 59 to second procedures that are not bundled into the primary procedure. As this book goes to print, CMS is developing additional HCPCS modifiers to further define situations in which modifier 59 would be used.

Key points:

Append modifier 59 to a secondary procedure code when

- the secondary procedure is a component of the first procedure
- there is no other modifier that more accurately describes the service and
- the secondary procedure meets the distinct and separate services definition.

See also: Medicare Physician Fee Schedule Database, multiple surgical procedures

Citations:

CMS, *Medicare Claims Processing Manual*, Pub 100-04, Chapter 12, Sections 40.6, 40.7, 40.8, http://www.cms.gov/Manuals/IOM/list.asp

OIG, *Use of Modifier 59 to Bypass Medicare's National Correct Coding Initiative*, November 2005, Pub. OEI-03-02-00771, http://oig.hhs.gov/oei/reports/oei-03-02-00771.pdf

https://www.cms.gov/Medicare/Coding/NationalCorrectCodInitEd/index.html

CMS document, MLN Matters article SE 1418 "Proper Use of Modifier 59"

Modifier 78—Unplanned Return to the Operating Room

Modifier 79—Unrelated Procedure during the Postoperative Period

Definition:

Modifier 78 is used to indicate that a return trip to the operating room or procedure room that is related to the original surgery was required during a global postoperative period. Modifier 79 is used to indicate that a return trip to the OR was required that was unrelated to the original surgery, during the global postoperative period.

Explanation:

The global postoperative period includes follow-up care for surgical procedures for the number of days indicated in the MPFSDB. If a return trip to the operating or procedure room is required during that postoperative period, the surgeon must use a modifier to be paid. The CPT® definition of modifier 78 is "Unplanned Return to the Operating/Procedure Room by the Same Physician or Other Qualified Health Care Professional Following Initial Procedure for a Related Procedure During the Postoperative Period: It may be necessary to indicate that another procedure was performed during the postoperative period of the initial procedure (unplanned procedure following initial procedure). When this procedure is related to the first, and requires the use of an operating/procedure room, it may be reported by adding modifier 78 to the related procedure." The definition of modifier 79 is "Unrelated Procedure or Service by the Same Physician or Other Qualified Health Care Professional During the Postoperative Period: The individual may need to indicate that the performance of a procedure or service during the postoperative period was unrelated to the original procedure. This circumstance may be reported by using modifier 79."

Codes: Modifiers 78 and 79 are used on procedures.

Coverage: All payers.

Billing and coding rules:

When using modifier 78, Medicare will pay only for the intra-operative portion of the code. CMS considers that the surgeon is already being paid for the preoperative and postoperative work from the original surgery. Use this modifier when a complication of the original procedure requires a return trip to the operating room. A new global period does not begin on the date of the second procedure.

Modifier 79 indicates that the second surgical procedure was performed by the same surgeon but was unrelated to the first surgical procedure. A different diagnosis should be submitted. A new postoperative period begins when a procedure is reported with modifier 79.

Related issues:

Medicare only pays for complications in the postoperative period if a return trip to the operating room is required.

Key points:

- Append modifier 78 to a surgical procedure during the global period for a return trip to the operating room that is related to the first surgery.
- Append modifier 79 to the surgical procedure during the global period for a return trip to the OR by the same surgeon that is unrelated to the original surgery.
- Modifier 58 is used for a staged or planned return trip to the OR.

See also: Global period, Modifier 58.

Citation:

CMS, *Medicare Claims Processing Manual*, Pub 100-04, Chapter 12, Section 40, http://www.cms.gov/Manuals/IOM/list.asp

Modifier PT—A Colorectal Cancer Screening Test Which Led to a Diagnostic Procedure

Definition:

Modifier PT is an HCPCS modifier used when a screening colonoscopy converts to a diagnostic or therapeutic procedure.

Explanation:

Modifier PT is described as "A colorectal cancer screening test which led to a diagnostic procedure." Use this modifier when during a scheduled colorectal screening procedure a physician performs a diagnostic or therapeutic service such as taking a biopsy or removing a polyp. This tells Medicare that although a diagnostic or therapeutic service is reported, the intent of the service was screening. The Medicare contractor will process the claim without a patient due co-pay or deductible.

Codes: Colorectal screening codes.

Coverage: Medicare. Private payers may prefer modifier 33.

Billing and coding rules:

The US Preventive Services Task Force (USPSTF) recommends certain screening procedures and immunizations, and gives these a rating. Any services that the USPSTF assigns an A or B rating are covered without co-pay or deductible for Medicare patients. Using modifier PT tells the Medicare contractor that this was such a service, even though a diagnostic or therapeutic service is reported.

Related issues:

Group private insurance policies sold after the implementation of the Affordable Care Act also have this provision.

Key points:

- Use modifier PT on Medicare claims when a colorectal screening test leads to a diagnostic or therapeutic service on that date.
- Use a screening diagnosis code and the code that supports the diagnostic or therapeutic service.

See also: Modifier 33

Citation:

Medicare Claims Processing Manual, Chapter 18, Sections 1.3 and 60
http://www.cms.gov/Regulations-and-Guidance/Guidance/Manuals/Downloads/
clm104c18.pdf

Multiple Endoscopic Procedures

Definition:

Medicare payment rules for multiple endoscopy procedures allow 100% of the primary procedure, plus the difference between the next highest valued procedure and the base procedure.

Explanation:

Physician payment for multiple endoscopies do not follow the usual multiple surgical payment rule. Payment is based on the family of endoscopy codes performed. Medicare and most insurers pay for the base payments in the family of codes only once. This means that for subsequent endoscopic procedures, the payment for second and subsequent procedures is small.

Codes: Endoscopy codes.

Coverage: Medicare and most other payers.

Billing and coding rules:

These codes are identified in the Medicare Physician Fee Schedule Database, by a three in field 21. When billing for multiple endoscopies, check the National Correct Coding Initiative (NCCI) edits. The base procedure in each family of codes is bundled into more complex codes in the series and may not be billed with the higher complexity code with any modifier. These are indicated as separate procedures in the CPT® book.

Many carriers do not require modifier 51 on the subsequent endoscopic procedures. Although applying modifier 51 meets the CPT® coding rules, check with your carrier and third-party payers before using it. If the second endoscopic procedure meets the criteria of a different or separate procedure, such as a different lobe or procedure performed at a different surgical session, apply the modifier 59 to the second procedure.

Related issues:

The reimbursement for secondary endoscopic procedures is low.

Key points:

- Check the NCCI edits for bundled procedures.
- Bill primary procedure with no modifier.
- Do not bill the diagnostic base procedure in a family of codes when billing more complex codes in that family.

- Bill secondary procedures with a modifier 51—or with no modifier if so instructed by your carrier or third-party payer.
- Bill secondary procedures that meet the criteria of a separate and distinct service with a 59 modifier.

See also: Multiple surgical procedures, modifier 51, modifier 59.

Citations:

CMS, *Medicare Claims Processing Manual*, Pub 100-04, chapter 12, Section 40.6, http://www.cms.gov/Manuals/IOM/list.asp

https://www.cms.gov/Medicare/Coding/NationalCorrectCodInitEd/index.html

Multiple Surgical Procedures

Definition:

Surgeons are paid at 100% of the fee schedule amount for the primary surgical procedure, and at 50% for the second to fifth surgical procedure performed at the same surgical session.

Explanation:

Billing for multiple surgical procedures performed at the same session depends on bundling rules, NCCI edits, correct modifier use, and relative value units (RVUs). To bill successfully for providing multiple surgical services on the same day, the physician needs to understand all of these coding rules.

Codes: Surgical procedures.

Coverage: All payers.

Billing and coding rules:

When performing multiple surgical procedures, physicians should code the major procedure with no modifier. The major procedure is the procedure with the highest relative value units in the Medicare Physicians Fee Schedule Database. Additional procedures, which are not component codes of the major procedure, are reported with modifier 51. Although it is correct coding, not all payers and carriers require modifier 51.

   Additional procedures which are components of the first procedure and do not meet the criteria for being distinct and separate are not submitted on the claim form. These are bundled or included in the payment for the primary procedure. When an additional procedure is a component and meets the criteria for being distinct and separate, use modifier 59.

   According to the *Medicare Claims Processing Manual*, bilateral surgeries are surgeries performed on both sides of the body by the same surgeon during the same session on the same day. If the surgical definition of the service is bilateral or says "unilateral or bilateral," the multiple surgery rules do not apply. Payment is already based on the service as a bilateral service. If the code description is "bilateral" the claim should not be submitted with the bilateral modifier. Bilateral surgeries are paid at 150% of the physician's fee schedule amount.

Related issues:

When using modifier 59 to bill for the second procedure, be sure that the second procedure meets the criteria of a distinct, separate service. Distinct and separate means that the service was provided at a different session or patient encounter; on a different organ or site; on a separate lesion; or for a different incision, excision, or injury. Do not apply it to the second service if it is not a component code of the first. Do not use it to bypass NCCI edit if the second service does not meet the criteria of the distinct and separate.

Key points:

Use this procedure when submitting claims for multiple surgical procedures.

1. List all codes for the procedures performed.
2. Note whether the procedures were performed via the same compartment, incision, site, organ system, lesion, injury, during the same session, and by the same surgeon. If all are the same, note "same." If any of the above are different, note "different."
3. Check the RVUs for each procedure and note them next to the code. The code with the highest RVU is the primary procedure; the others are secondary procedures. Note the primary procedure.
4. Check the NCCI edits. If the secondary procedures are component codes of the primary procedures, and the procedure is the same (as indicated above), bill only the primary procedure.
5. If the secondary procedures are not component codes of the primary procedure, and the procedure is the same (as defined above), bill the primary procedure with no modifier and the secondary procedures with modifier 51. This indicates that multiple procedures were performed that fall into the category of "same" as indicated above.
6. If the secondary procedures are component codes of the primary procedure, but the procedure meets the difference criteria above (different session, compartment, lesion, injury, etc.), bill the primary procedure with no modifier and bill the secondary procedures with modifier 59.

See also: Multiple endoscopy procedures, Medical Physician Fee Schedule Database, modifier 50, modifier 51, modifier 59.

Citations:

CMS, *Medicare Claims Processing Manual*, Pub 100-04, Chapter 12, Sections 40.6, 40.7, 40.8, http://www.cms.gov/Manuals/IOM/list.asp

OIG, http://oig.hhs.gov/oei/reports/oei-03-02-00771.pdf (for the modifier 59 report from the OIG)

National Correct Coding Initiative (NCCI)

Definition:

The National Correct Coding Initiative (NCCI) Edits are CMS developed edits for the purpose of processing claims correctly and controlling improper or incorrect payments to providers.

Explanation:

The NCCI edits define payment policies to ensure uniform and correct payments to physicians and other healthcare providers. Services denied by Medicare due to NCCI edits may not be billed to Medicare beneficiaries, whether or not the provider obtained an ABN. Mutually exclusive edits are services that could not be provided together: a hysterectomy could not be performed both vaginally and abdominally. These types of edits are now displayed as column 1/column 2 edits. Certain modifiers allow a claim to bypass the NCCI edits, and these modifiers must be applied correctly to insure both revenue collection and compliance.

If carriers apply these edits uniformly, it reduces the variation in how claims are processed amongst carriers. There are also Medically Unlikely Edits, for units and anatomy that are not published.

Codes:

The NCCI edits include thousands of code pairs and are updated quarterly.

Coverage:

These are Medicare edits, but they are adopted by many other carriers. Some insurers develop their own edits.

Billing and coding rules:

All practices need to check the NCCI edits for services they perform when the same physician provides more than one service to the same patient on the same day. There are three ways to do this. The first is to download a free copy of these edits from the CMS web site. Practices no longer have to buy the NCCI edits. The web site address is in the citation section of this entry. A second easier way to use the NCCI edits is to buy a computer program or subscribe to a web site that allows the user to type in the procedure codes and check for bundling edits or mutually exclusive code pairs. All of the major commercial providers of coding books have single and multi-user computer systems available. There are web-based subscription programs available. The NCCI edits on paper are notoriously difficult to use and understand, so a computer-based system is preferable. The third option available to some practices is a claims editor integrated with a billing system. This is a terrific option if available from the a practice management or clearinghouse vendor.

The introduction to the NCCI manual defines what services are included in surgical procedures. This includes vascular and airway access and cardiac monitoring, anesthesia provided by the physician who is performing the service, non-diagnostic biopsies, exploration of the surgical field, access through abnormal tissue, incision and opening, treatment of complications such as bleeding, unless a return to the operating room is required. This introduction provides an important overview to NCCI. A copy of it can be downloaded in the manual section from CMS. It is titled, "NCCI Policy Manual for Part B Medicare Carriers."

The modifiers that bypass the NCCI edits include modifier 22, unusual procedural service, modifier 25, significant, separately identifiable service, modifier 50, bilateral procedure, modifier 58, staged or related procedure by the same physician during the post-op period, and modifier 59, separate procedure.

Related issues:

The global surgical package also defines services that are considered part of the global payment.

Key points:

- Download and read the introductory material to the NCCI edits. These word-based chapters explain the theory behind the edits for each chapter.
- Check for bundled procedures and mutually exclusive procedures prior to billing the services provided, when more than one service is provided by the same physician, on the same date, to the same patient.
- Consider using a computer-based program to check NCCI edits.
- Do not bill the patient, with or without an ABN, for procedures denied because they are mutually exclusive or bundled.
- Review the rules related to modifiers 25 and 59.

See also: Modifier 25, modifier 59, multiple surgical procedures

Citations:

https://www.cms.gov/Medicare/Coding/NationalCorrectCodInitEd/index.html

Medicare Claims Processing Manual, Pub 100-04, Chapter 23 http://www.cms.gov/Manuals/IOM/list.asp

National Coverage Determinations (NCDs)

Definition:

National Coverage Determinations (NCDs) are statements of Medicare policy that describe whether a medical service or supply is covered by Medicare and in what circumstances it is covered.

Explanation:

Medicare pays for services that it considers "reasonable and necessary for the diagnosis or treatment of an illness or injury." CMS bases its determinations on evidence-based medicine, and it allows physicians and other members of the public to comment on proposed NCDs.

Codes:

There is a long list of diagnostic services and other procedures covered by these policies.

Coverage:

These are Medicare policies. Private payers develop their own policies related to the medical necessity, indications and frequency of providing services.

Billing and coding rules:

The CMS web site has a list of NCDs and Local Coverage Determinations that can be searched by keyword or accessed alphabetically. Each NCD notes the publication number, manual section, version, effective and implementation dates, benefit categories (such as diagnostic tests, physician services, and durable medical equipment) and coverage topics (such as diagnostic tests and durable medical equipment). The service is described and the covered clinical indications for the service or test are listed. The NCDs also describe non-covered indications. For some policies, frequency limitations are listed. The policy lists cross-references to CMS transmittals to the manuals, and to transmittal links.

In a fee-for-service environment, payers typically pay for a service based on CPT® codes but the service can be denied based on the diagnosis code. The diagnosis code shows the medical necessity for the service. Submitting a claim for which there is an NCD when the patient does not have a covered indication will result in a denial. Using NCDs allows the practice to discuss non-covered services with the patient prior to providing the service. The practice then has the opportunity to obtain an Advance Beneficiary Notice (ABN) from the patient, if the physician and patient want to continue with the service. The patient will be financially liable for the service if an ABN is properly executed.

Related issues:

Medicare and all third-party payers use medical necessity as a key determinant in deciding whether to pay or deny a claim. NCDs are a way that Medicare has attempted to standardize coverage indications and limitations for services, using evidence-based medicine. Physician practices and individual patients do not always agree with these decisions.

Key points:

- Research NCDs for services provided in the practice.
- If a patient does not have a covered indication for the service as indicated in the NCD, inform the patient that it is non-covered before providing the service or before prepping the patient for the service.
- Properly execute an ABN if the patient wishes to proceed.
- Educate your staff about ABNs and assign responsibility for explaining coverage to the patient and obtaining an ABN.
- If possible, build these rules into your claims processing systems so the posting staff is alerted at the time of posting if the diagnosis code and the procedure code do not match.

See also: Advance Beneficiary Notice, Local Coverage Determinations, medical necessity

Citations:

CMS overview: http://www.cms.gov/medicare-coverage-database/overview-and-quick-search.aspx

Alphabetical listing: http://www.cms.gov/medicare-coverage-database/indexes/ncd-alphabetical-index.aspx

New Patient

Definition:

A new patient is a patient who has not received any professional service from the physician or from another physician of the same specialty in the same group within the past three years. The CMS definition is of a new patient is, "Interpret the phrase "new patient" to mean a patient who has not received any professional services, i.e., E/M service or other face-to-face service (e.g., surgical procedure) from the physician or physician group practice (same physician specialty) within the previous 3 years. For example, if a professional component of a previous procedure is billed in a 3-year time period, e.g., a lab interpretation is billed and no E/M service or other face-to-face service with the patient is performed, then this patient remains a new patient for the initial visit. An interpretation of a diagnostic test, reading an x-ray or EKG etc., in the absence of an E/M service or other face-to-face service with the patient does not affect the designation of a new patient."

Explanation:

Some Evaluation and Management services are divided into new and established patient visits. A new patient is defined by time limits, by the specialty of the physician, and by the physician's membership in the group. A professional service is any face-to-face medical, surgical, or diagnostic service.

Codes: Office/outpatient visits, domiciliary or rest home visits, home visits, and preventive medicine services.

Coverage:

The CPT® definition states "exact same subspecialty" instead of specialty, but payers follow the CMS rules.

Billing and coding rules:

Bill an established patient visit if the patient has been seen by that physician or by another physician of the same specialty in the same group within the past three years. Although the CPT® book uses the phrase, "exact same subspecialty" in the definition of a new patient, CMS and third-party payers only recognize certain specialties when determining if a patient is new or established. The payers use CMS's two-digit specialty code designations, not the more specific National Uniform Claim Committee's 10-digit healthcare provider taxonomy codes, which recognizes additional specialties and subspecialties.

Here are some "what if" scenarios.

What if a physician changes groups within the same town? A physician who sees a patient and then joins a new group in the same town will bring many of his or her own patients to the new practice. If the physician has provided a professional service in the past three years, that patient is considered an established patient visit in the new office.

What if a physician sees a patient for the first time in the hospital, and the patient follows up in the office? A physician who sees the patient in the hospital and then sees the patient for the first time in his or her office should bill for an established patient visit, because the physician had a recent face-to-face service with the patient in the hospital.

What about covering for another physician? A physician who is covering for another physician in the group of the same specialty, even if he or she is not seeing the patient personally, will also bill for an established patient visit if the patient is considered established to the first physician. This is a CPT® rule.

The CPT® book states that a qualified health care professional—their term for advance practice nurses and physician assistants—is working in a practice, consider them to be of the same specialty when determining if a patient is new or established. Be careful when there are multiple locations of the same specialty in the same group. Under Medicare guidelines, pay for physicians in a group of the same specialty as if they were one physician, even if they practice in a different location. This definition of group membership has a large impact on the definition of new patient visits. However, physicians of different specialties may both see a patient and bill an office visit service on the same date. Similarly, preventive care services are divided into new and established patient visits, and the same rules apply.

Related issues:

Many Evaluation and Management (E/M) services are not categorized as new and established, including consultations, inpatient and observation hospital services, emergency department visits, and nursing home services. Some of these have initial and subsequent designations, and some do not.

Key points:

- Bill for physicians in a group of the same specialty as if they were one physician.
- A new patient is a patient who has not had a professional service from that physician or from another physician of the same specialty within the past 3 years.
- Be careful when billing for physicians of one specialty who practice in multiple locations.

See also: Consultations.

Citation:

> CMS, *Medicare Claims Processing Manual*, Pub 100-04, Chapter 12, Sections 30.6.5 and 30.6.7, http://www.cms.gov/Manuals/IOM/list.asp

Nurse Visit

Definition:

The lowest level Evaluation and Management (E/M) established patient visit provided by a nurse or medical assistant in the physician office can be billed as a nurse visit.

Explanation:

Established patient visits have five levels of service. The lowest level of service, 99211, may be billed by a nurse or other clinical staff member. The CPT® book tells us that this service may not require a face-to-face visit from a physician. There are no explicit documentation requirements for this code, but the service must be documented in the medical record.

Code: 99211.

Coverage:

A practice must meet the requirements for incident to services to bill a nurse visit to a Medicare patient. Other payers' coverage varies.

Billing and coding rules:

The most important billing rule to remember for Medicare patients is that to bill with code 99211, the service must meet the criteria for incident to rules. Other payers' rules will vary, of course. Like all medical services, a nurse visit must be medically necessary. Practices should not use this code automatically in addition to another service on a routine basis, such as an allergy injection. Injection codes 96372 and 99211 may never be reported on the same calendar date. Do not use 99211 when the service provided is more accurately described by another CPT® code, such as vaccine administration or venipuncture. The nurse who sees the patient should document in the progress note section of the chart, not just on a flow sheet. The nurse who performs the service should provide a separate note, which would typically include the reason for the visit, a brief history, exam (such as vital signs), and a brief assessment and plan. The plan may describe the patient's medications or any discussion with the physician.

A blood pressure check is a typical reason for a nurse visit on a Medicare patient. For non-Medicare patients, a nurse might address a new problem covered under an office protocol, such as a urinary tract infection. This would not be appropriate on a Medicare patient, because new problems do not meet the criteria of incident to services.

Related issues:

Sometimes, practices want to bill a nurse visit on the same day that a patient sees a physician or a Non-Physician Practitioner (NPP). No payers will pay for a 99211 in addition to an office visit on the same day.

Key points:

- For Medicare, the service must meet incident to requirements.
- The nursing staff member should sign and date the note for that visit.
- Do provide separate documentation.
- Do not automatically bill a nurse visit with another service, such as an allergy injection.
- Remember, medical necessity is the key to providing all medical services.
- Do not bill a nurse visit in place of another service which is more accurately described by another CPT® code, such as an injection or venipuncture.

See also: Documentation Guidelines, incident to services.

Citation:

CMS, *Medicare Claims Processing Manual*, Pub. 100-04, Sections 20.3, 30.5, 30.6.4, http://www.cms.gov/Manuals/IOM/list.asp

Nursing Facility Visits

Definition:

Nursing facility visits are Evaluation and Management (E/M) services performed in a skilled nursing facility or a nursing facility.

Explanation:

Nursing facility codes may be used in place of service 31 for patients in a Part A covered skilled nursing facilities. They can be used in place of service code 32 for patients in non-Part A covered skilled nursing facility beds, in non-covered skilled nursing facilities, or in nursing facilities.

Who may bill for nursing home codes? Physicians and NPPs may bill for nursing facility codes, but only a physician may bill for initial nursing facility care (99304–99306) in a skilled nursing facility (SNF). After the initial service has been provided, a physician and an NPP may alternate providing subsequent nursing facility care (99307–99310). Although it does not make much sense from the code descriptions, an NPP may provide the subsequent nursing facility care to a patient before the physician performs and bills for the initial nursing facility care.

In a nursing facility, (as differentiated from a skilled nursing facility) NPPs who are not employed by the nursing facility may bill for the initial service as long as that service is within their scope of practice, meets their state law, and meets collaboration and supervision requirements. An NPP in a nursing facility may bill for all of the subsequent nursing facility visits.

There are two levels of nursing facility discharge: one for a discharge that takes the provider 30 minutes or less and one for a discharge that takes more than 30 minutes to complete. This is the total time of the discharge, not the face-to-face time with the patient.

The code for an annual assessment is now 99318.

Codes:

99304–99306	Initial nursing facility care
99307–99310	Subsequent nursing facility care
99315–99316	Nursing facility discharge services
99318	Other nursing facility services (annual assessment)

Coverage: Visits covered based on patient status in the nursing facility.

Billing and coding rules:

The physician must bill for the initial admission service in the skilled nursing facility. After that, the physician and the NPP may alternate visits. NPPs may bill for subsequent nursing facility visits before or after the physician has performed the admission. This can be useful when the physician does not get to the nursing facility within the first day or two to see the patient. The NPP can bill for a subsequent nursing facility visit even before that admission was performed.

In a nursing facility, the NPP may perform all subsequent nursing visits.

Although it is usually difficult to successfully bill for two E/M services in one day, a physician may be paid for both a discharge from the hospital and an admission to the nursing facility on the same date. However, the physician may not use the discharge service as the admission and bill for both. The physician must see and discharge the patient in the hospital to bill 99238 or 99239, and then the physician must have a face-to-face service with the patient in the skilled nursing facility to bill for the initial skilled nursing facility service.

Bill for an initial nursing facility service or discharge on the calendar date of the visit even if it does not correspond with the admission or discharge date.

Related issues:

How frequently must the physician or NPP see a patient who is in a skilled nursing facility? A visit is required within 30 days of the admission, every 30 days within the first 90 days of care, and every 60 days after that. These are not CPT® or Part B Medicare rules but are part of the facility's conditions of participation with Medicare.

If the clinician is asked to see a patient for a medical problem, that visit may be used as one of the required visits; the clinician need not provide the medically necessary service one day and then do the mandated review service the day after that. Skilled nursing services may not be billed as incident to or shared visits. If an NPP performs the service in a nursing facility, bill under the NPP provider number, not the physician's provider number.

Key points:

- All nursing facilities are per day codes by CPT® definition. Only one nursing home visit is paid in a single day.
- The physician must bill for the admission to the skilled nursing facility.
- An NPP may bill for an admission to the nursing facility in certain, very limited, situations. The NPP must not be an employee of the nursing facility and it must be within that NPP's scope of practice, allowed by state law, and covered under applicable supervision requirements.

- After the initial service in the skilled nursing facility the MD and the NPP may alternate visits.
- A physician may delegate all nursing facility visits to an NPP.
- The place of service billed is based on the designation of the patient: a skilled nursing facility is Place of Services (POS) 31 and a nursing facility is POS 32.
- Providers must meet frequency requirements for nursing facility patients.
- A medically necessary visit or an annual assessment can count as one of the mandated visits according to the frequency requirements.
- Bill for NPP Services under their own provider number, not under the physician's provider number.

See also: Consolidated nursing home billing.

Citation:

CMS, *Medicare Claims Processing Manual*, Pub 100-04, Chapter 12, Section 30.6.13, http://www.cms.gov/Manuals/IOM/list.asp

Osteopathic Manipulative Treatment

Definition:

Osteopathic manipulative treatment (OMT) is "a form of manual treatment applied by a physician or other qualified healthcare professional to eliminate or alleviate somatic dysfunction and related disorders."[1]

Explanation:

OMT is used to relieve low back pain, somatic dysfunction, and other musculoskeletal abnormalities and injuries. There are over 20 different types of manual treatment techniques, but whichever technique is used the same codes are reported. These include physical manipulations, deep pressure and traction and spinal adjustments.

Codes:

98925–98929 osteopathic manipulative treatment. The code selected depends on the number of body regions that were treated. (1–2, 3–4, 5–6, 7–9, 9–10) The number of lesions does not affect the coding. If three lesions are treated in one region, count that as one body region treated. Bill only one OMT code per encounter.

Coverage:

The service has a status indicator of active from Medicare and is covered by most commercial insurers. Some payers may implement frequency limitations.

Billing and coding:

It is critical that physician who is providing the treatment documents which body regions were treated and by what method. The body regions defined in the CPT® book are: head, cervical, thoracic, lumbar, sacral, pelvic, lower extremities, upper extremities, rib cage, abdomen and viscera.

One of the most vexing problems when providing this service is getting paid for a separate and distinct E/M service on the same calendar day. According to CPT, an E/M service may be provided on the same day as OMT and reported with modifier 25. CPT® goes on to say that the E/M service and OMT maybe the result of the same symptoms or condition, and thus a different diagnosis is not required according. Many practices find that commercial payers require different diagnoses if both are reported and that for established patients an E/M service is denied on the same day as an OMT treatment. If the note

---

[1] Current Procedural Terminology, 2018 American Medical Association

starts with, "Patient presents for an OMT treatment," the payer will likely deny a separate E/M service.

For an initial evaluation, it is easier to be paid for both services. The clinician evaluates the condition, which includes a physical exam, and in the course of the evaluation decides to perform an OMT treatment. Documenting the results of the exam, and the clinical thinking that shows that OMT is required based on the history and exam is helpful in supporting both services. Documenting the somatic dysfunction shows the medical necessity for the treatment.

Payers often have a list of covered indications, and these can be searched for and found on their websites. For OMT, these will typically be related to somatic disorders. Non-musculoskeletal conditions will not serve as the medical necessity for OMT for most private payers.

Related issues:

Documentation is key when reporting OMT and an E/M service on the same day. Review payer policies carefully to avoid denials.

Key points:

- Document the number of regions and the type of OMT provided for each region.
- For initial services, report both an E/M service and OMT when the documentation shows a separate evaluation of the condition, prior to the decision to perform OMT. Use modifier 25 on the E/M service.
- For follow up services, report a separate E/M when the documentation shows that a separate evaluation of the condition was made, prior to the decision to perform the treatment.
- When planned, repeat OMT is documented as the reason for the visit, report only the OMT.
- Check payer policies for coverage.

See also: Modifier 25

Citation:

CPT® Assistant , October 2009, Volume 19, Issue 10, pages 10–11.

Pelvic and Breast Clinical Exam

Definition:

A pelvic and clinical breast exam is a physical screening service described by Medicare using code G0101, cervical or vaginal screening, pelvic and clinical breast exam.

Explanation:

Medicare was created for the treatment of illness or injury and routine services are statutorily excluded from Medicare coverage. Over the years, however, Congress has passed provisions that allow Medicare to pay for certain screening services within diagnosis code and frequency limitations. Medicare also pays for a small number of immunizations. The pelvic and breast exam is one example of a covered screening service.

In addition to paying for the pelvic and breast exam, Medicare will pay for obtaining and preparing the specimen for a PAP smear using code Q0091. Codes G0101 and Q0091 are covered annually for high-risk patients, and every other year for low-risk patients.

There are specific exam elements required, as outlined below.

Codes:

G0101 Cervical or vaginal cancer screening; pelvic and clinical breast examination

Q0091 Screening Papanicolaou (PAP) smear; obtaining, preparing and conveyance of cervical or vaginal smear to laboratory

Coverage: Medicare

Billing and coding rules:

Medicare pays for a pelvic exam every two years for low-risk patients and annually for high-risk patients.

High risk factors for cervical or vaginal cancer include the following:

1. Early onset of sexual activity (under 16 years of age)
2. Multiple sexual partners (five or more in a lifetime)
3. History of sexually transmitted diseases (STDs)
4. Fewer than three negative pap smears within the previous seven years
5. Diethylstilbestrol-exposed (DES-exposed) daughters of women who took DES during pregnancy

G0101 (Cervical or vaginal screening; pelvic and clinical breast exam) is used to bill for the exam. This exam should include seven of the 11 elements below and must include a breast exam:

- Inspection and palpation of the breasts for masses, lumps, tenderness, asymmetry, or nipple discharge
- Digital rectal exam

Pelvic exam, including the following:

- External genitalia
- Urethral meatus
- Bladder
- Urethra
- Vagina
- Cervix
- Uterus
- Adnexa/parametria
- Anus and perineum

This service may be done on the same day as a covered wellness visit, or on the same day as an E/M service (office visit), or on the same day as a non-covered physical exam. If done on the same day as an E/M service, attach the 25 modifier on the office visit.

HIGH RISK DIAGNOSIS CODES	
Code	**Description**
Z72.51	High-risk heterosexual behavior
Z72.52	High-risk homosexual behavior
Z72.53	High-risk bisexual behavior
Z77.29	Contact with and (suspected) exposure to other hazardous substances
Z77.9	Other contact with and (suspected) exposures hazardous to health
Z91.89	Other specified personal risk factors, not elsewhere classified
Z92.89	Personal history of other medical treatment

LOW RISK DIAGNOSIS CODES	
Code	Description
Z01.411	Encounter for gynecological examination (general) (routine) with abnormal findings
Z01.419	Encounter for gynecological examination (general) (routine) without abnormal findings
Z12.4	Encounter for screening for malignant neoplasm of cervix
Z12.72	Encounter for screening for malignant neoplasm of vagina
Z12.79	Encounter for screening for malignant neoplasm of other genitourinary organs
Z12.89	Encounter for screening for malignant neoplasm of other sites

Related issues:

An Advance Beneficiary Notice (ABN) is required if you perform the G0101 and Q0091 at a greater frequency than is allowed. Be sure to properly execute the ABN with specific reasons why you believe Medicare might not cover the service. Commercial payers will often pay the Q0091 code. The service described by G0101, however, is part of an age and gender appropriate physical exam. It would be incorrect to bill G0101 on the same day as you bill the preventive medicine services to commercial patients.

Key points:

- These codes are diagnosis code specific. Using a general examination code will result in a denial.
- These codes have specific frequency limitations.
- Obtain an ABN if either the diagnosis or the time limit code requirements are not met.
- Make sure to document seven of the 11 bullets for the pelvic and clinical breast exam.

See also: Preventive medicine services, preventive medicine services for Medicare patients, Advance Beneficiary Notice.

Citations:

https://www.cms.gov/Medicare/Prevention/PrevntionGenInfo/medicare-preventive-services/MPS-QuickReferenceChart-1.html#PAP

CMS, *Medicare Claims Processing Manual*, Pub 100-04, Chapter 18. http://www.cms.gov/Manuals/IOM/list.asp

Preoperative Exams

Definition:

Primary care providers and specialty providers are often asked to provide preoperative clearance before a patient may go to surgery. These services are billed with E/M codes.

Explanation:

Once the decision for surgery is made and the patient is scheduled for surgery, the surgeon may not report an E/M service for the purpose of a preoperative history and physical even when that history and physical (H&P) is mandated by the hospital or surgery center. A visit for the purpose of an H&P and informed consent is not separately billable but is part of the global payment for the surgery. An E/M service that meets the requirements of modifier 25 or 57 may be separately reported.

A primary care physician (PCP) or other specialist may report an E/M service if the surgeon requests medical clearance prior to surgery. These medically necessary services are covered by Medicare and other third parties. They should be reported with the correct category of code. In the office, this is a consult or new or established patient visit.

Codes: E/M services

Coverage: All payers

Related issues:

E/M services prior to a screening colonoscopy are never paid by Medicare. A medically necessary E/M service is payable for diagnostic colonoscopy prior to the procedure.

Key points:

- A consult for a preoperative clearance for payers that still pay for consults may only be billed if all of the requirements necessary for a consultation are met: a request from another healthcare professional, the rendering of an opinion, and a report returned to that healthcare professional.
- There are diagnosis codes for preoperative exams.

See also: Consultations, global surgical package, modifier 25, modifier 57, and category of code chart

Citation:

CMS, *Medicare Claims Processing Manual*, Pub 100-04, Chapter 12, Section 30.6.6 and Section 40, http://www.cms.gov/Manuals/IOM/list.asp

Preventive Medicine Services

Definition:

A preventive medicine service includes an age and gender appropriate history and exam, anticipatory guidance, risk factor reduction, provision of or referral for immunizations, and screening diagnostic tests.

Explanation:

Well visits, annual exams, physical exams: These are the words we use to describe the physician office component of preventive medicine services. These visits are defined as new and established patients, and age groups. They include an age and gender appropriate comprehensive history and comprehensive exam. The CPT® book tells us that these comprehensive histories and exams are not the same as defined by the documentation guidelines. That is, the history does not require four items on the history of the present illness, 10 systems reviewed, and all of the patient's past family, social, and medical history. Instead, the history is composed of a review of systems and past family, social, and medical history that is relevant to the patient's age and gender. For a child, this history will include developmental history. Similarly, the exam required is not the eight organ system comprehensive exam required for high level E/M codes.

The CPT® book suggests that clinicians consult their specialty societies, the US Preventive Services Task Force (USPSTF), and the CDC for recommendations about what to include in these services, as well as what screening tests and immunizations to provide.

Codes: 99381–99397

Coverage:

Annual physical exams do not have an A or B rating from the US Preventive Services Task Force (USPSTF), and as defined by CPT®, are not covered by Medicare. Medicare does pay for wellness exams, including the Welcome to Medicare Visit and the Initial and Subsequent Wellness visits. Most commercial payers cover a preventive medicine service and pay for it without applying a co-pay or deductible.

Billing and coding rules:

Most private pay policies allow annual billing of a preventive medicine service after the age of two. Prior to age two, babies and toddlers are seen more often. Follow the new patient rule to determine whether the patient is new or established, and then select the code based on the patient's age.

Provide and document an age and gender appropriate history and physical exam. Also, provide anticipatory guidance and risk factor reduction appropriate to the patient's age and gender. This includes recommendations for immunizations and screenings. These recommendations to patients are part of the definition of preventive medicine services. Clinicians may bill separately, however, for performing these screening tests. Also bill separately for the administration of immunizations and for the vaccine, if the vaccine was purchased by the practice.

Some practices want to bill separately for G0101, pelvic and breast exam, when billing for a code in the preventive medicine series. This is bundled into the preventive medicine codes for commercial patients. (Medicare rules are rules unto themselves and are discussed elsewhere in this book.)

The CPT® book includes immunization administration codes for vaccines. CMS has HCPCS codes for the administration of the immunizations it covers. These codes are defined by the method of administration, whether or not the physician provided counseling about the vaccines, and the age of the patient.

What about addressing a patient's medical problems on the same day as a preventive medicine service? Can a clinician be paid for two E/M services on the same day, the preventive medicine service and the office visit? According to the CPT® book, if a physician or NPP addresses an acute or chronic medical problem that requires significant extra work to perform key elements of the history, exam and medical decision making, the clinician can bill an office visit. The CPT® book tells us to bill an office visit with a 25 modifier on the same day as a preventive medicine service. This is correct coding, but is can be difficult to collect from third parties. The problem-oriented E/M service may be patient due, and this can cause patient complaints. Many Medicaid programs will only pay for one service in a day, and will select the lower paying code as the one to pay! However, billing staff should track their success in collecting for these services.

Related issues:

Diagnosis coding is critical in preventive medicine service, particularly for screening tests and immunizations.

Key points:

- Preventive medicine services include an age/gender appropriate history and exam, anticipatory guidance and risk factor reduction, referral for screening tests, and provision of immunizations.
- Most commercial policies cover these without a co-pay or deductible.

- Bill for administration of vaccines and for the vaccine if the practice bought the serum.
- Coding rules allow a physician to bill for an office visit and a preventive medicine service on the same day, using a modifier 25 on the office visit. Do this when significant extra work was performed to diagnose or treat a patient's illness. The E/M service may be patient due.
- Be careful about diagnosis coding. Non-specific diagnosis coding may result in denials.

See also: New patients, pelvic and breast exam, preventive medicine for Medicare patients, welcome to Medicare, wellness visits for Medicare patients

Citation:

Agency for Healthcare Research and Quality, http://www.ahrq.gov/clinic/uspstfix.htm (U.S. Preventive Task Force web site).

Preventive Medicine Services (Medicare)

Definition:

Medicare was developed for the care of sick and injured beneficiaries, and was not intended to cover preventive medicine services.

Explanation:

Over the years, Congress has passed many laws that pay for screening or preventive services. Annual physical exams are not covered by Medicare. However, the Health Care Reform Act of 2010 added in coverage for an annual wellness visit. CMS developed HCPCS codes to report wellness visits because they do not correspond to existing CPT® definitions. In addition, the Affordable Care Act mandated that any preventive services that the US Preventive Services Task Force (USPSTF) gives an A or B rating will be covered for Medicare beneficiaries. Medicare also pays for a "Welcome to Medicare" visit.

Codes:

99381–99397 for preventive medicine services are not covered.
G0402—Welcome to Medicare visit
G0438 and G0439 for wellness visits
Many HCPCS codes for covered screening services

Coverage:

By Medicare statute. Covered screening services have gender, diagnosis and frequency limits.

Billing and coding rules:

When billing for the covered screening and immunizations provided to Medicare patients, there are often HCPCS codes used in place of the CPT® codes.

Related issues:

The CMS web site provides an interactive chart of covered preventive medicine services. This lists the specific CPT®, HCPCS, and ICD-10 codes that are covered for Medicare patients and the frequency of coverage. The citation is at the end of this entry.

Key points:

- Medicare does pay for many screening tests and immunizations. Use the specific HCPCS codes and diagnosis codes for those to prevent denial for these services.

See also: Preventive medicine services; "Welcome to Medicare" visit, pelvic and breast exam, wellness visits

Citations:

Medicare Claims Processing Manual, Pub 100-04, Chapter 18

https://www.cms.gov/Medicare/Prevention/PrevntionGenInfo/Medicare-Preventive-Services/MPS-QuickReferenceChart-1.html#PAP

Prolonged Services—Face-to-Face

Definition:

Prolonged services are defined as Evaluation and Management (E/M) services that take the provider 30 minutes more than the typical time for that code. Prolonged services codes are add-on codes to specific E/M services. This article describes face-to-face prolonged codes.

Explanation:

Many E/M services have typical times established for each code. These are listed in the CPT® book and include new patient visits, established patient visits, initial hospital services, subsequent hospital services, observation services, nursing facility services, and consults. There is no typical time defined for emergency department visits or most preventive medicine services.

Physicians and NPPs may use the add-on codes with specific E/M codes to indicate that the face-to-face time spent exceeded the typical time for that code by 30 minutes or more.

Medicare requires start and stop time although this is not a CPT® rule. When reporting prolonged services for Medicare patients, start and stop times are required. For prolonged services reported with office or outpatient services, the prolonged service is face-to-face time for both CPT® and Medicare rules. For prolonged services reported with inpatient services, CPT® states that unit time may be counted, but Medicare states that the additional time must be face-to-face with the patient.

Codes:

99354–99357 for prolonged services with face-to-face contact

Coverage:

Prolonged service codes are typically covered for face-to-face services. Some payers may request records.

Billing and coding rules:

Never bill these codes alone. Always add them on to the appropriate E/M services when you submit your claim. The time provided does not need to be continuous, but only provider time counts. A practice may not bill for staff time under prolonged services codes.

For example, a patient with asthma presents to the practice with wheezing and shortness of breath. The physician orders a nebulizer treatment, and the patient is in the office treatment room for 60 minutes. A staff member is with the patient for all of that time. The physician, however, spent 10 minutes with the patient in doing an assessment and ordering the treatment and has checked on the patient twice during the hour. The total physician time is 20 minutes. In this case, it is incorrect to bill a prolonged services code.

Document provider time in the medical record. "I spent a total of 60 minutes with the patient in face-to-face service today." (See Prolonged Services Code Chart, next page.) Medicare requires start and stop times, not simply a statement of the total time.

What about visits that are entirely counseling, for which no history and exam are documented? This might be the case in a situation when a patient returns to talk about a known diagnosis and the treatment options. Medicare says that if the visit is entirely counseling, use the highest level code in that category of code before using prolonged services. For example, a patient returns to an oncologist to discuss the treatment options for breast cancer, and the entire visit is spent in that discussion. The visit category is established patient visit, and the total face-to-face visit time was 80 minutes. First, look at the typical time for the highest code in that category, 99215. It is 40 minutes. Then, look at the chart to see what the threshold time is to bill the prolonged services code. It is 70 minutes or 30 minutes more than the typical time. In this case, bill 99215 and 99354.

Can prolonged services be used for a second hospital visit on the same day, by the same physician or that physician's same-specialty partner? Yes, in rare circumstances. The initial visit must have time documented. The second visit must have the time documented as well. For Medicare, the second visit, on which the prolonged services code is based, must be for face-to-face, not unit, time and must be documented with the start and stop time. Most prolonged hospital services take place on the unit but not necessarily the bedside. The Medicare rules are more stringent than CPT® rules in requiring the prolonged service to be exclusively face-to-face with the patient.

			Threshold time
	Typical time	**Threshold time**	**to bill codes**
Code	**for code**	**to bill 99354**	**99354 & 99355**
New patient, office			
99201	10	40	85
99202	20	50	95
99203	30	60	105
99204	45	75	120
99205	60	90	135
Established patient, office			
99212	10	40	85
99213	15	45	90
99214	25	55	100
99215	40	70	115
Office and outpatient consults			
99241	15	45	90
99242	30	60	105
99243	40	70	115
99244	60	90	135
99245	80	110	155
Home visits			
99341	20	50	95
99342	30	60	105
99343	45	75	120
99344	60	90	135
99345	75	105	150
99347	15	45	90
99348	25	55	100
99349	40	70	115
99350	60	90	135

The table is titled **Prolonged Services Codes**.

Related issues:

Match the prolonged services codes with the E/M service for which they are covered. Prolonged services are add-on codes. Never bill an add-on code on its own.

Key points:

- Document the total provider time in the medical record; Medicare requires start and stop times.
- Document the medical necessity for the additional time in providing the services. Why did it take so long to see this patient?
- Use these with their companion E/M code and not for procedures or for any other E/M codes.

See also: Time-based codes, Prolonged Services—non-face-to-face, Prolonged Services for preventive medicine (HCPCS).

Citation:

CMS, *Medicare Claims Processing Manual*, Pub 100–04, Chapter 12, Section 30.6.15, http://www.cms.gov/Manuals/IOM/list.asp

Prolonged Services—Non-Face-to-Face Codes: 99358 and 99359

Definition:

In 2017, Medicare recognized and began paying for non-face-to-face prolonged services using existing Current Procedural Terminology (CPT®) codes.

Explanation:

These codes are for prolonged services by the billing physician and non-practitioner physician (NPP) when provided in relation to an Evaluation and Management (E/M) service or other face-to-face service on the same or different day as an E/M service. If the clinician meets half of the threshold time for the prolonged service without face-to-face contact (31 minutes), use code 99358. Follow CPT® rules for the service.

Codes:

99358: Prolonged Evaluation and Management service before and/or after direct patient care; first hour

+ 99359 each additional 30 minutes (List separately in addition to code for prolonged services.)

Coverage:

These are valid CPT® codes. Although commercial insurers are not required to follow CMS policy, many do.

Billing and coding rules:

These E/M services allow a physician or NPP to be paid for non-face-to-face work related to a face-to-face E/M service. The two services do not have to be performed on the same day. The example given in the CPT® book is for extensive record review. However, other coordination services could meet the requirements.

Because Medicare is following CPT® rules for these services, the CPT® rules related to time are in effect. I always think this is a "through the looking glass rule." However it is a well-established CPT® principle. For a service defined with a time component, the clinician must meet over half of the time stated. In the introduction in your CPT® book under the heading of time, it indicates the following:

"A unit of time is attained when the mid-point is passed. For example, an hour is attained when 31 minutes have elapsed (more than midway between zero and sixty minutes). A second hour is attained when a total of 91 minutes have elapsed."

In the case of these non-face-to-face prolonged services that means that code 99358 may be reported when 31 minutes have been spent. To report the add-on code 99359, 76 minutes would need be spent in the non-face-to-face prelaunch services work. There is no provision or splitting this work over to calendar dates. This time rule does not relate to the stated times for E/M services.

Neither CPT® nor Medicare in the 2017 final rule limits the specialty of physician or NPP who can perform these services. Although CMS discusses it in the section related to improving payment accuracy for primary care, there is no prohibition for other specialties using these codes. These codes could be relevant for any physician or NPP who needs to review extensive records prior to a patient visit when the time reaches the 31-minute threshold.

Of course, document time in the medical record and briefly describe the work completed.

Related issues:

CMS uses these existing CPT® codes as a way to support primary care physicians (PCPs) and the cognitive work done in managing the care of patients. However, the codes are not limited to PCPs.

Key points:
- This service may be provided on the same day or on a different day than the face-to-face service.
- This is for the work of the physician or NPP, not staff.
- It is for extensive time in addition to seeing the patient and must relate to a service for a patient where direct face-to-face patient care has occurred or will occur and be part of ongoing patient management.
- Code 99358 is not an add-on code. That is it can be reported on the day when no other service is provided.
- Code 99359 is an add-on code to code 99358.
- The prolonged time need not be continuous but must occur on one day.
- CPT® tells us not to report these services during the same month as complex chronic care management (codes 99487, 99489) or during the service time of transitional care management (codes 99495, 99496).
- You cannot double count the time for these non-face-to-face prolonged services codes and time spent in certain other activities represented by specific CPT® codes. However, the list of CPT® codes are mostly those which have

a status either non-covered or bundled by Medicare. (Care plan oversight: codes 99339, 99340, 99374–99380; medical team conferences: 99366–99368, online medical evaluations: 99444, or other non-face-to-face services with more specific codes and no upper limit in the CPT® codes.)

See also: Chronic care management, transitional care management

Citation:

https://www.cms.gov/Outreach-and-Education/Medicare-Learning-Network-MLN/MLNMattersArticles/downloads/mm5972.pdf

Prolonged Services: Healthcare Common Procedural Coding System (HCPCS) Codes for Preventive Care

Definition:

The Centers for Medicare and Medicaid Services (CMS) has developed two new HCPCS codes to be used with a short list of Medicare preventive services. These codes are prolonged services, used in addition to the preventive service, when the total of face-to-face time of the visit meets the threshold beyond the typical intra-service time.

Explanation:

A frequently asked question is what to do if a Medicare wellness visit or welcome to Medicare visit is unusually lengthy. Prior to 2018, the only alternative was to add a problem-oriented visit if that describes the extra time. But if the additional time for the Medicare preventive service was all related to prevention, there was no additional reimbursement for the primary care clinician.

Codes:

G0513: Prolonged preventive service(s) (beyond the typical service of the primary procedure) in the office or other outpatient setting requiring direct patient contact beyond the usual service; first 30 minutes (listed separately in addition to code for preventive service)

G0514: Prolonged preventive service(s) (beyond the typical service of the primary procedure) in the office or other outpatient setting requiring direct patient contact beyond the usual service; each additional 30 minutes (listed separately in addition to code for preventive service)

Coverage: Fee-for-service Medicare

Billing and coding rules:

Use these codes only with Medicare covered preventive medicine services. CMS developed these codes to report only with Medicare-covered preventive services when the clinician provides a prolonged Medicare-covered preventive service. These codes may only be billed with Medicare covered preventive services, and the patient will not be charged a co-pay or deductible. They are used to report and be paid for the additional time when the total time exceeds that intra-service work time for the preventive service. Prior to this, CMS had not published typical times for wellness visits or for the welcome to Medicare visit. CMS has developed chart that lists the typical intra-service time for our use.

CMS follows Current Procedural Terminology (CPT®) rules for the existing prolonged services codes. It follows CPT® rules when determining time for face-to-face prolonged services in addition to Evaluation and Management (E/M) codes, critical care, and physical therapy. Here is the CPT® rule:

> "A unit of time is attained when the midpoint is passed. For example, an hour is attained when 31 minutes elapsed (more than midway between zero and sixty minutes). The second hour is attained when a total of 91 minutes have elapsed."

Although CMS does not mention this in the 2018 Final Rule, it seems reasonable to assume that CMS will follow the same rules for these prolonged services codes as they do for prolong services codes with other E/M services.

Of course, check with your individual Medicare Administrative Contractor (MAC) to see how they are interpreting this rule.

Don't add a problem-oriented E/M code. The Final Rule does not say this directly, but in reading between the lines, I believe that if three codes are on the claim form (wellness visit, prolonged, and problem-oriented), codes G0513 and G0514 will be denied.

At the time of this book's printing, it's unclear if a practice will need to append modifier 25 to code G0513 or G0514 or to the preventive exam, or if they are considered add-on codes and will not need a modifier.

Use G0513 and G0514 with these services:

Code	Brief description	Intra-service time of physician, NP, PA	Threshold to bill G0513	Threshold to bill G0513 & G0514
G0402	Welcome to Medicare visit	30	46	76
G0438	Wellness visit, initial	30	46	76
G0439	Wellness visit, subsequent	25	41	71
Q0091	Obtaining screen pap smear	16	32	62
G0101	Ca screen; pelvic/breast exam	10	26	56

G0104	Ca screen; flexible sigmoidscope	17	33	63
G0105	Screening colonoscopy, high-risk individual	30	46	76
G0121	Screening colonoscopy, not high-risk individual	30	46	76
G0296	Visit to determine lung cancer screening eligibility	15	31	61
16 minutes added for first prolonged services code; CPT® rule for time				

Related issues:

This continues CMS's support for primary care practices and addresses concerns of primary care physicians (PCPs).

Key points:

- Use these HCPCS codes only with the Welcome to Medicare visit (G0402), Initial and subsequent wellness visits (G0438, G0439), and the other services listed in the chart.
- Document the additional time in the medical record
- This is the time of the physician or non-practitioner physician (NPP), not staff time.

See also: Welcome to Medicare, Medicare Wellness Visits

Citation:

https://www.cms.gov/Medicare/Medicare-Fee-for-Service-Payment/PhysicianFeeSched/PFS-Federal-Regulation-Notices-Items/CMS-1676-F.html

Psychiatric Collaborative Care Management Services 99492, 99493, 99494

Definition:

In 2018, these Current Procedural Terminology (CPT®) codes replaced the HCPCS codes for Collaborative Care Management, Behavioral Health Integration (CoCM-BHI) that were developed by CMS in 2017. The Healthcare Common Procedural Coding System (HCPCS) codes G0502, G0503 and G0504 are no longer active.

Explanation:

These are new codes to describe the work performed in primary care practices for patients with behavioral health issues. CMS intended this as part of its support for primary care physicians (PCPs). The PCP directs the work of a behavioral health care manager (BHM) in consultation with a psychiatric physician and psychiatric non-physician practitioner (NPP). This recognizes the work and time of practitioners and staff in caring for patients with behavioral conditions outside of an Evaluation and Management (E/M) visit. These services require an initiating visit by a physician or NPP who can perform E/M services as part of his or her scope of practice. (CPT® uses the term qualified healthcare professional.)

These patients "typically" have a newly diagnosed condition, according to the 2018 CPT® book but may also have an existing condition and need help in engaging in treatment or have not responded to standard treatment.

When CMS developed the (now deleted) HCPCS codes in 2017, they said this in their Final Rule:

> "A specific model for BHI, psychiatric CoCM typically is provided by a primary care team consisting of a primary care provider and a care manager who works in collaboration with a psychiatric consultant, such as a psychiatrist. Care is directed by the primary care team and includes structured care management with regular assessments of clinical status using validated tools and modification of treatment as appropriate. The psychiatric consultant provides regular consultations to the primary care team to review the clinical status and care of patients and to make recommendations."

Codes:

99492: Initial psychiatric collaborative care management, first 70 minutes in the first calendar month of behavioral health care manager activities, in consultation with psychiatric consultants and directed by the treating physician or other qualified health care professional, with the following elements:

- Outreach to and engagement in treatment of a patient directed by the treating physician or other qualified health care professional
- Initial assessment of the patient, including administration of validated rating scales, with the development of an individualized treatment plan
- Review by the psychiatric consultant with modifications of the plan if recommended
- Entering patient in a registry and tracking patient follow up and progress using the registry, with appropriate documentation, and participation in weekly caseload consultation with the psychiatric consultant
- Provision of brief interventions using evidence-based techniques such as behavioral activation, motivational interviewing, and other focused treatment strategies

99493: Subsequent psychiatric collaborative care management, first 60 minutes in a subsequent month of behavioral health care manager activities, in consultation with a psychiatric consultant, and directed by the treating physician or other qualified health care professional, with the following required elements:

- Tracking patient follow up and progress using the registry, with appropriate documentation;
- Participation in weekly caseload consultation with the psychiatric consultant;
- Ongoing collaboration with and coordination of the patient's mental health care with the treating physician or other qualified health care professional and any other treating mental health providers;
- Additional review of progress and recommendations for changes in treatment, as indicated, including medications, based on recommendations provided by the psychiatric consultant;
- Provision of brief interventions using evidence-based techniques, such as behavioral activation, motivational interviewing, and other focused treatment strategies;
- Monitoring of patient outcomes using validated rating scales, and relapse prevention planning with patients as they achieve remission of symptoms and/or other treatment goals and are prepared for discharge from active treatment;
- Relapse prevention planning with patients as they achieve remission of symptoms and/or other treatment goals and are prepared for discharge from active treatment.

+99494: Initial or subsequent psychiatric collaborative care management, each additional 30 minutes in a calendar month of behavioral health care manager activities, in consultation with a psychiatric consultant, and directed by the treating physician or other qualified health care professional (List separately in addition to code for primary procedure.) (Use G0504 in conjunction with codes 99492, 99493.)

These care management services are for patients with a psychiatric diagnosis.
- Services provided under the supervision of a PCP by a behavioral health manager
- Services in consultation with a psychiatric clinician who can prescribe medications
- Time of the behavioral health manager in a calendar month
- For patients with behavioral health conditions who "could have newly diagnosed conditions, need help in engaging in treatment, have not responded to standard care delivered in a non-psychiatric setting, or require further assessment and engagement" before referral to psychiatry

An episode of care begins with the start of this intervention and ending with
- The attainment of targeted treatment goals, which typically results in the discontinuation of care management services and continuation of usual follow up with the treating physician or other qualified health care professional
- Failure to attain targeted treatment goals culminating in referral to a psychiatric care provider for ongoing treatment
- Lack of continued engagement with no psychiatric collaborative care management services provided over a consecutive 6-month calendar period (break in episode)
- A new episode starts after a break of six months

Coverage:

These are active CPT® codes, but check with commercial payers about coverage.

Billing and coding rules:

These describe psychiatric collaboration of care for CoCM-BHI. These codes provide payment to physicians and NPPs in a primary care practice to direct a behavioral care manager in collaboration with a consulting psychiatrist, psychiatric nurse practitioner (psychiatric NP), or psychiatric physician assistant (psychiatric PA). Care is directed by the primary care team using structured management and regular assessments, validated tools, and modifications of the treatment plan as needed. These are services provided by the BHM at the direction of the physician and NPP in a calendar month.

It requires that the behavioral health manager consult with the psychiatric consultant who is a psychiatric physician and NPP who is able to prescribe the full range of psychiatric medications. This is not separately reimbursed to the psychiatrist but is part of the payment for the collaboration of care model. That is, the psychiatrist would look for payment from the primary care practice with which he or she is consulting. CMS believes they have valued these services to include this payment.

CPT's coding tip for these services states that the physician or qualified health professional (NP/PA) may personally perform these services, but time cannot be double counted for any other service. Time spent coordinating care for a patient in the Emergency Department (ED) may be counted but may not report time spent if the patient is admitted to inpatient or observation status.

These services are billed by the physician or NPP for services provided by the BHM.

The behavioral health manager and psychiatrist need not be employees; they can be contracted with the primary care practice.

Diagnosis codes:
- New or established behavioral health condition
- Specific codes not established by CMS
- Condition that warrants referral to the BHM

Behavioral health care manager (BHM)
- CPT® defines this as a clinical staff member with a masters/doctoral level education or "specialized training in behavioral health"
- Could be a professional who is eligible to bill Medicare, but this is not required
- May be an employee or contracted agent
- Must be able to see the patient face-to-face when needed but does not need to be in the same location as PCP
- Services are provided both face-to-face and non-face-to-face
- The behavioral health manager may provide psychotherapy services to the patient and report these separately but may not double count the time spent doing care management and psychotherapy

Service requirements
- Weekly consultation between the BHM and psychiatric consultant
- Psychiatric consultant must be physician or NPP who is able to prescribe full range of psychiatric medications
- Psychiatric consultant advises and makes recommendations for psychiatric care and medications, differential diagnosis, treatment strategies, and management of complications

- The medical record should document the components described in the code, including engagement with the patient, the initial assessment, and the rating scales used in the assessment. The individualized treatment plan and discussion with the psychiatric consultant needs to be documented. The BHM must enter the patient into a registry that allows for tracking patient follow up and progress.
- The BHM should document any interventions made with the patient. Because these are time-based codes, the time of the individual activities will need to be documented.
- The PCP may provide medically necessary E/M services during the period.
- The psychiatrist or psychiatric NP/PA could perform needed assessments and bill for those but are not required to see the patient as part of CoCM services.
- The psychiatrist may bill for a psychiatric evaluation but may not double count any time or activities in care management and the psychiatric evaluation.

Related issues:
- A code exists for care management of a patient with behavioral conditions that has less difficult requirements. Chronic Care Management (CCM) codes could also be used for patients with behavioral and other medical conditions.

Key points:
- Care directed by primary care physician and NPP
- An initiating E/M visit is required
- The patient must have a behavioral health diagnosis
- The plan, implementation and changes to the plan need to be documented
- Time spent in the activities by the behavioral health manager must be documented in the medical record
- Behavioral health manager enters patient into a registry and tracks progress
- The continuing involvement and direction of the physician and NPP should be documented
- Weekly consultation with psychiatrist or psychiatric NP/PA who can prescribe a full range of psychiatric medications
- General supervision for service, not direct; physician and NPP does not need to be in the office with the behavioral health manager when services is provided

See also: chronic care management, care management for behavioral conditions

Citation
   CPT® 2018

Reviewing Medical Records

Definition:

Physicians and Non-Physician Practitioners (NPPs) routinely review voluminous medical records for new and established patients.

Explanation:

The care of a patient requires both primary care and specialty clinicians to review prior medical records. This review can be time consuming. Documenting the information discovered in this review counts in the calculation of the amount of data reviewed for medical decision making for an E/M service and may—but does not always—increase the level of medical decision-making when deciding on the level of service. However, beginning in 2017, CMS recognized non-face-to-face prolonged services codes. These may be used for record review that is greater than 30 minutes, and is not typical pre and post visit work.

Codes: None.

Coverage: None.

Billing and coding rules:

Reviewing medical records is part of the preparatory and follow-up work of a paid medical service, but payers do not reimburse separately for this service. Reviewing medical records and documenting the information found there is one of the data points considered in the amount of data reviewed for an Evaluation and Management service. Here is what the documentation guidelines say about that:

> DG: Relevant findings from the review of old records, and/or the receipt of additional history from the family, caretaker, or other source to supplement that obtained from the patient should be documented. If there is no relevant information beyond that already obtained, that fact should be documented. A notation of "Old records reviewed" or "additional history obtained from family" without elaboration is insufficient.

The widely used Marshfield Clinic audit sheet for selection assigns two data points for this review. Not all carriers follow that guideline. With other data, this sometimes results in a higher level of medical decision-making. Medical decision-making is only one of the three key components in selecting an E/M service, so a higher level of medical decision-making might result in a higher E/M code.

Related issues:

Physicians and NPPs perform many non-reimbursable services in the course of their day. Reviewing prior medical records is one of these. CMS considers this work part of the pre-work and post work for a billable service.

Key points:

- Payers do not offer separate reimbursement for reviewing old medical records.
- Time spent before or after the visit may not be included in the time of the visit, if time is used to select the E/M code in the office.
- Document what additional information was obtained from the old record.
- This data review may result in a higher level of medical decision making for an E/M code.

See also: Telephone calls, care plan oversight, care plan oversight for Medicare patients, time-based codes, prolonged services, non-face-to-face.

Citation:

CMS Documentation Guidelines, http://www.cms.gov/Outreach-and-Education/Medicare-Learning-Network-MLN/MLNEdWebGuide/EMDOC.html

Shared Visits (Medicare)

Definition:

Shared visits are E/M services that are shared or split between a physician and a qualified Non-Physician Physician Practitioner (NPP) in the inpatient or outpatient setting or in the Emergency Department (ED).

Explanation:

If a physician and an NPP each provide part of an E/M service in the hospital (inpatient/outpatient/ED), the visit may be billed as a shared visit, using the physician provider number. This allows the practice to bill for the service under the physician provider number and be paid for the service at 100% of the physician fee schedule. (Shared services done in the physician's office must meet incident to rules.)

Codes: E/M codes.

Coverage: These are Medicare rules.

Billing and coding rules:

In a shared visit, both the physician and the NPP have a face-to-face service with the patient, and both document their part of the visit in the medical record. The physician must see the patient and document some clinically relevant portion of the note. This does not need to be extensive or repetitive but must be more explicit than "Seen and agree." The physician note, which is typically less extensive than the NPP note, should show that the physician saw the patient and participated in the care in a meaningful way. For example, the physician might note the following: "Saw patient. Agree with Mr. Scully's plan. We'll follow her labs again tomorrow and hopefully can discharge her." Or the physician might note the following: "Saw patient. Agree with Mr. Scully's history and plan. Her lungs sound clearer to me and she reports that she has less shortness of breath at night."

If the documentation shows that both the physician and NPP had face-to-face services with the patient, and both have documented something of clinical relevance, bill the service under the physician's provider number. Add together the documentation elements from both notes to select the level of service. If the physician did not see the patient, but provided supervision or advice to the NPP, bill the service under the NPP provider number. NPPs are paid at 85% of the physician fee schedule.

Because shared visits in the office must meet the incident to guidelines, shared visits may only be billed for established patient visits in the office. If the visit meets the incident to guidelines, it may be billed under the physician provider number whether or not the physician saw the patient and provided part of the care.

Related issues:

Groups with a large number of inpatients often use NPPs as a way of managing their care. The physician can spend part of the day in the hospital, but return to the office to see patients there for most of the day. The NPP stays at the hospital, writes the longer notes, and does the management the rest of the day. This not only saves the physician time in documentation, but keeps them from the interruption of repeated phone calls with lab results, requests for new orders, etc. Many practices find this an effective way to manage patients. Hospitalist groups also often use NPPs and report services under the shared services rules.

Key points:

- This is a Medicare rule. Check with commercial payers for their rules.
- Both the physician and the NPP must document a face-to-face service with the patient.
- The physician must document a clinically relevant portion of the history, exam or medical decision making. Writing something like "Seen and agree" is insufficient.
- Shared visits are allowed in the hospital in inpatient and outpatient departments and in the ED. Shared visits are only allowed in the office if they meet incident to requirements.
- Bill shared visits under the physician provider number and combine the documentation from both providers to select the level of service.

See also: Incident to services.

Citation:

CMS, *Medicare Claims Processing Manual*, Pub. 100-04, Chapter 12, Section 30.6.1, http://www.cms.gov/Manuals/IOM/list.asp

Smoking Cessation Counseling

Definition:

There are CPT® codes for smoking cessation counseling, based on time.

Explanation:

Smoking-related illnesses account for significant preventable morbidity and death. These codes may be added on to an E/M code when the time spent in counseling the patient to quit smoking is explicitly documented.

Codes:

99406 Smoking and tobacco use cessation counseling visit; intermediate, greater than three minutes up to 10 minutes.

99407 Smoking and tobacco use cessation counseling visit; intensive greater than 10 minutes.

Coverage:

Most private payers cover smoking cessation using the CPT® codes. The HCPCS codes for smoking cessation were deleted.

Commonly used diagnoses:

Use a code from category F17, nicotine dependence. Some payers will require another diagnosis code, for the condition that is worsened by smoking, such as COPD, diabetes or heart disease.

Billing and coding rules:

The smoking cessation service may be provided on the same day as an E/M service as long as there are two significant, separately identifiable services provided. For example, a clinician might treat a patient's diabetes and chronic obstructive pulmonary disease and provide smoking cessation counseling at the same visit. Append modifier 25 to the E/M service.

Medicare will cover eight sessions in a 12-month period when using the HCPCS codes for an asymptomatic patient. After one year has elapsed, another eight sessions are allowed for the beneficiary. Keep in mind that this is not a service that is allowed eight times per provider, but eight times per patient by any provider.

The diagnosis code submitted with the claim should reflect the patient's condition that is adversely affected by tobacco use. Smoking cessation services that take fewer than three minutes are part of the E/M service and are not separately billable.

Whenever time is used to select a CPT® code or an HCPCS code, document the time spent in smoking cessation, exclusive of the E/M service.

Related issues:

An Advance Beneficiary Notice (ABN) will be required if the physician provides the service more frequently than is allowed by Medicare. An ABN will also be needed if multiple physicians are providing the service to one patient and they have surpassed the number of services that the patient is allowed.

Key points:

- Remember to document time in the medical record when providing smoking cessation.
- Use the diagnosis code related to the patient's illness for which the smoking cessation counseling is provided.

See also: Time-based codes.

Citations:

CMS, *Medicare Claims Processing Manual*, Pub 100-04, Chapter 32, Section 12, http://www.cms.gov/Manuals/IOM/list.asp

Medicare National Coverage Determination, 210.4, Smoking and tobacco-use Cessation Counseling: For more detail on multiple sessions and documentation requirements, *see* Medicare Downloadable Brochure at: http://www.cms.gov/Outreach-and-Education/Medicare-Learning-Network-MLN/MLNMattersArticles/downloads/MM7133.pdf

Teaching Physician Rules Based on Time

Definition:

The teaching physician rules for CPT® codes based on time allow an organization to bill only for the time spent and documented by the attending physician, not the resident. The terms "attending physician" and "teaching physician" are used interchangeably in this entry.

Explanation:

Procedure codes determined on the basis of time are billable in a teaching physician setting based solely on the time spent and documented by the attending physician. Although the resident may see the patient with the teaching physician before or after the teaching physician service, only the time spent by the attending physicians counts in code selection.

Codes:

Following are the codes from the *Medicare Claims Processing Manual*, which are based on time.

- Individual medical psychotherapy (CPT® codes 90832–90853)
- Critical care services (CPT® codes 99291–99292)
- Hospital discharge day management (CPT® codes 99238–99239)
- E/M codes in which counseling and/or coordination of care dominates (more than 50 percent) of the encounter, and time is considered the key or controlling factor to qualify for a particular level of E/M service
- Prolonged services (CPT® codes 99354–99359)
- Care plan oversight (HCPCS codes G0181–G0182).

Coverage: Teaching physician rules are Medicare rules.

Billing and coding rules:

For psychiatric time-based codes, the requirement for the attending physician, not the psychologist, may be met by concurrent observation of the service by use of a one-way mirror or video equipment. Audio equipment does not meet the requirement.

For all other services, the attending physician must personally document the time he or she spends providing the care.

For E/M codes based on time, the attending physician should document the total time of the visit, note that the visit was more than 50% counseling, and describe the nature of the counseling.

Related issues:

Time-based codes require time to be documented in the medical record, not just the billing record.

A resident is defined by Medicare as a physician enrolled in an approved graduate medical education program. Append modifier GC to these services.

Key points:

- To use a time-based code, the attending physician must personally be present for the time of the service provided.
- The attending physician must personally document in the medical record the time spent providing the service.
- Use modifier GC on claims for teaching physician services. This modifier does not affect payment but tells the carrier that these were services performed using the teaching physician rules.

See also: Teaching physician rules for critical care, teaching physician rules for procedures, teaching physician E/M services, teaching physician rules for medical students, time-based codes, critical care.

Citation:

CMS, *Medicare Claims Processing Manual*, Pub. 100-04, Chapter 12, Section 100, http://www.cms.gov/Manuals/IOM/list.asp

Teaching Physician Rules for Critical Care Services

Definition:

These rules govern the provision of critical care services in a teaching institution when those services are billed by an attending physician, and a resident has participated in the patient's care. The terms "attending physician" and "teaching physician" are used interchangeably in this entry.

Explanation:

In a teaching facility, attending physicians, fellows, residents, and medical students all participate in the care of a patient. Medicare has specific rules and policies describing which services must be personally performed and documented by the attending physician to bill for the services under the attending physician's name.

Critical care codes are time-based codes. Although a resident participates in the care of a critically ill patient, only the attending physician's time is counted when reporting the service.

Codes: 99291–99292.

Coverage: These are Medicare rules.

Billing and coding rules:

Only count the attending physician's critical care time. The attending physician must personally document all of the requirements for critical care. Documentation should state that the patient is critically ill, that the attending physician provided critical care treatment to that patient, and how much time the attending physician spent in providing care. The resident's note will supplement this entry about the patient's condition and treatment, but the resident physician's time cannot be counted in critical care billing. It would be insufficient to write "Seen and agree" by the attending physician with the resident's note.

Apply modifier GC to the critical care code.

Related issues:

Review the requirements for critical care billing. The patient must be critically ill, critical care services must be provided to the patient, and time must be documented in the medical records.

Key points:

- The attending physician must provide critical care services to the patient and document that the time spent providing critical care was 30 minutes or more to meet the threshold to bill 99291.
- The attending physician must legibly sign the critical care note.
- It should be clear what service the attending physician provided.
- Time spent in teaching does not count as critical care time billable to Medicare.
- Apply the GC modifier to services provided under the teaching physician rules.

See also: Teaching physician rules for E/M services, teaching physician rules with primary care exception, teaching physician rules for surgical procedures, procedures, teaching physician rules for medical students, teaching physician rules for time-based care, critical care.

Citation:

CMS, *Medicare Claims Processing Manual*, Pub 100-04, Chapter 12, Section 100, http://www.cms.gov/Manuals/IOM/list.asp

Teaching Physician Rules for Evaluation and Management Codes

Definition:
There are a specific set of rules for the attending physician to comply with to bill for Evaluation and Management (E/M) services provided jointly by a resident and an attending physician, and reported under the attending physician's provider number. The terms "attending physician" and "teaching physician" are used interchangeably in this entry.

Explanation:
The teaching physician rules for the supervision of residents define a resident as an intern, resident, or fellow enrolled in an accredited graduate medical education program. A medical student is never considered to be a resident. An attending physician may bill for the services provided jointly with a resident if the attending physician sees the patient, performs a critical or key portion of the E/M service, and participates in the patient's management. The attending physician may see the patient jointly with the resident and be physically present for the entire session, or may see the patient at a different time from the resident physician. The attending physician's services may partially overlap with the resident or may be performed at a different time on the same calendar date.

The attending physician must personally document his or her participation in the patient's care and link his or her work with the resident note, following specific Medicare guidelines.

Codes: E/M services.

Coverage: Medicare, and other payers.

Billing and coding rules:
The first requirement for the attending physician to bill for an E/M service done jointly with a resident physician is that the attending physician must see the patient. The attending physician must participate in the care of the patient by performing the key elements/critical portions of the E/M service, and then documenting the service in a way that links the attending physician's note and the resident's note.

The attending physician must have a face-to-face contact with the patient to bill for the service. The teaching physician must personally document that they performed the service or were physically present with the resident who performed the service and must document their own participation in the care of the patient.

Here are other examples of linking statements that meet the criteria:

- For initial hospital services: "I performed a history and physical examination of the patient and discussed his management with the resident. I reviewed Dr. Resident's note and agree with the documented findings and plan of care. I would consider increasing his dosage of Lasix."

- For a subsequent hospital visit: "Day three. I saw and evaluated the patient. I agree with the assessment and plan as documented in Dr. Cardiology Resident's note."

- For a subsequent hospital visit: "Internal medicine attending note: I saw and examined the patient. I agree with the resident's note. The heart murmur is louder, so I suggest that we consult Cardiology for a possible echo."

- Initial hospital service or subsequent care: "I was present with Dr. Resident during the entire history and exam. We discussed the case and I agree with the findings and plan as documented in Dr. Resident's note."

- Subsequent care: "I saw the patient with the resident and agree with Dr. Resident's findings and plan."

- Initial or follow-up visit: "I saw and evaluated the patient. Discussed with Dr. Resident and agree with the findings and plan as documented in Dr. Resident's note."

Here are examples of attending physician statements that do not meet the criteria: "Seen and agree" and "Agree with resident's note."

The *Medicare Claims Processing Manual* addresses the situation that arises when the patient is admitted by a resident on one calendar date and the attending sees the patient the next day. From Chapter 12, Section 100:

> "When a medical resident admits a patient to a hospital late at night and the teaching physician does not see the patient until later, including the next calendar day:

- The teaching physician must document that he/she personally saw the patient and participated in the management of the patient. The teaching physician may reference the resident's note in lieu of re-documenting the history of present illness, exam, medical decision making, review of systems and/or past family/social history provided that the patient's condition has not changed, and the teaching physician agrees with the resident's note.

- The teaching physician's note must reflect changes in the patient's condition and clinical course that require that the resident's note be amended with further information to address the patient's condition and course at the time the patient is seen personally by the teaching physician.

- The teaching physician's bill must reflect the date of service he/she saw the patient and his/her personal work of obtaining a history, performing a physical, and participating in medical decision making regardless of whether the combination of the teaching physician's and resident's documentation satisfies criteria for a higher level of service. For payment, the composite of the teaching physician's entry and the resident's entry together must support the medical necessity of the billed service and the level of the service billed by the teaching physician."

Related issues:

Services provided under the primary care exception rule have different requirements.

Medical students are not considered residents and their services may not be billed by the attending physician. Medical students may only document a review of systems and the family, medical, and social history for an Evaluation and Management service.

NPP students, that is nurse practitioner students or physicians assistant students, are not considered residents, and the services for these students may not be billed by an attending physician or an NPP.

Append modifier GC to these services.

Key points:

- The attending physician must document that the patient was seen that day and his or her own participation in the patient's care through medical decision making.
- The Medicare claims processing manual specifically states that entries such as "seen and agree" or "seen with a resident and agree with above note" are insufficient. The documentation must reference the resident's note, show physical presence of the attending physician and document participation in the care. Supervision alone is insufficient.
- The attending physician does not need to repeat an entire portion of the note to bill for the service.
- The resident may not document the attending physician's presence or participation for E/M services.
- The attending physician must document his or her own participation.
- Append modifier GC to these services.

See also: Teaching physician rules for E/M services, teaching physician rules for a primary care exception, teaching physician rules on procedures, teaching physician rules for medical students, teaching physician rules for time-based care, critical care.

Citation:

CMS, *Medicare Claims Processing Manual*, Pub 100-04, Chapter 12, Section 100, http://www.cms.gov/Manuals/IOM/list.asp

Teaching Physician Rules for Medical Students

Definition:

Medical students are not residents, and their services may not be billed using the teaching physician rules. NPP student services are not payable by Medicare under the teaching physician rules. The terms "attending physician" and "teaching physician" are used interchangeably in this entry.

Explanation:

Medicare has developed specific rules for documenting and reimbursing teaching physician services. Medical students are not defined as residents and may not be billed using these rules.

Codes: All.

Coverage: These are Medicare rules but are typically followed by other payers.

Billing and coding rules:

For an E/M service, a medical student, physician assistant student, or nurse practitioner student may only document a review of systems and the medical, family, and social history. Many organizations have the student document a full note, but the student's note may not be the basis of the billing. The attending physician or resident must perform and document all other portions of the E/M service, including the chief complaint, history of present illness, exam, assessment, and care plan. If a medical student documents a review of systems and the family medical history, the attending physician should indicate that he or she has reviewed this information.

A procedure performed by a medical student may not be billed.

Related issues:

For an E/M service, a medical student may only document what another staff person in the physician office can document: a review of systems and the family/medical/social history. NPP student services are not payable. It is insufficient to countersign a note by a student and write "seen and agreed."

Key points:
- Medical students and NPP students may only document reviews of systems and past medical/family/social histories. It is permissible to allow the student to document more of the note, but the billing may not be based on their note.
- Medical student services are not covered by the teaching physician rules.

See also: Teaching physician rules for E/M services, teaching physician rules for primary care exceptions, teaching physician rules for surgical procedures, teaching physician rules for time-based care.

Citations:

CMS, *Medicare Claims Processing Manual*, Pub 100-04, Chapter 12, Section 100, http://www.cms.gov/Manuals/IOM/list.asp

CMS, http://www.cms.gov/Outreach-and-Education/Medicare-Learning-Network-MLN/MLNEdWebGuide/EMDOC.html

AAMC, https://www.aamc.org/download/253810/data/medicalstudent documentationinanehr.pdf

Teaching Physician Rules for Primary Care Exception

Definition:

The teaching physician rules allow carriers to pay for physician claims furnished by residents without the presence of an attending physician when the services meet the requirements for the primary care exception. The terms "attending physician" and "teaching physician" are used interchangeably in this entry.

Explanation:

Graduate medical education (GME) programs that plan to use the primary care exception billing rules must attest in writing, and keep in their own files, a statement that all of the requirements are being met. The services must be furnished in the outpatient department of a hospital or other ambulatory care center in which the time spent by residents are included in determining direct GME payments to the hospital by the fiscal intermediary.

The resident must have completed more than six months of residency to provide these services without the presence of an attending physician.

Codes: 99201–99203 and 99211–99213, G0402, Welcome to Medicare, G0438 and G0439, wellness visits.

Coverage: Medicare.

Billing and coding rules:

The teaching physician may supervise up to four residents at any one time under the primary care exception rule. During the time of the supervision, the teaching physician may not have any other responsibilities; must assume responsibility for those patients seen by the residents; must ensure that appropriate services are rendered; must review the history, exam, diagnosis, and plan with each resident during or immediately after each visit; and must document the extent of the review and care plan in the services furnished to each beneficiary.

The patients must consider the center to be their continuing source of healthcare. Residents must generally follow the same group of patients during their residency.

Residents may provide typical primary care services of acute or chronic problems. The *Medicare Claims Processing Manual* states that family practice, general internal medicine, geriatric medicine, pediatrics, and obstetrics/

gynecology are the specialties most likely to qualify for the primary care exception.

Bill for these services with modifier GE.

Related issues:

There are a limited number of services that may be reported under the primary care exception.

Key points:

- Organizations need to keep records on file showing that they qualify for the primary care exception. These do not need to be submitted to their fiscal intermediary or carrier, and pre-approval is not needed.
- An attending physician may supervise up to four residents at a time and have no other clinical responsibilities during this time period.
- The resident must have completed six months of an approved GME program to be eligible to bill under this rule.
- There are specific and limited services that may be reported under the primary care exception.
- The attending physician must document his or her supervision of the resident's care of the patient.
- Append modifier GE on claims submitted using the teaching physician rules.

See also: Teaching physician rules for E/M services, teaching physician rules procedures, teaching physician rules for medical students, teaching physician rules for time-based care.

Citation:

CMS, *Medicare Claims Processing Manual*, Pub 100-04, Chapter 12, Section 100, http://www.cms.gov/Manuals/IOM/list.asp

Teaching Physician Rules for Surgical Procedures

Definition:

The teaching physician rules for Medicare have specific rules regarding the performance of procedures by residents for the attending physician to bill for the service under the attending's provider number.

Explanation:

The teaching physician rules for Medicare require that the attending physician be present for the entire procedure for minor surgeries that take fewer than five minutes. Very few procedures take fewer than five minutes. For major procedures, the attending physician must be physically present for the critical or key portions of the procedure and must be immediately available to provide assistance during the remainder of the procedure. For endoscopy, the attending physician must be present from the introduction of the scope until its withdrawal. The terms "attending physician" and "teaching physician" are used interchangeably in this entry.

Codes: Surgical procedures.

Coverage: Medicare.

Billing and coding rules:

For a minor procedure or for endoscopy, the resident or nurse may document the attending physician's presence. For a single major procedure, the resident may document the attending's presence. If the attending is supervising two overlapping procedures, the attending must be present for the key and critical components of each and must document their own presence in the surgeries.

The teaching physician is responsible for the preoperative, operative and postoperative care, although the teaching physician may decide which postoperative visits require his or her presence.

An example of an attending physician statement which links to the resident note is "I was present for the critical key portions of the procedure and immediately available for the remainder of the procedure."

Minor procedures of fewer than five minutes duration require that the attending physician be present for the entire procedure.

For endoscopies, the attending physician must be personally present in the room for the entire viewing from when the scope is introduced until the scope is withdrawn. Viewing from a monitor is insufficient to allow the attending physician to bill for the endoscopy performed by a resident.

For major procedures, the attending physician must be physically present for the critical/key portions of the surgical procedure and must be immediately available to provide assistance during the entire procedure. For overlapping surgeries, the teaching physician must be present for the critical portions of each surgery. In addition, the teaching physician must personally document the key portions of both procedures. If the teaching physician leaves the operating room after key portions of the procedure to start another procedure, another physician must be available to intervene in the first case, should that be necessary. A resident does not qualify as a physician for this purpose. Indicate the name of the second surgeon in the note. If an attending physician is involved in supervising three overlapping surgeries, the attending physician may not bill for these concurrent surgical procedures.

Append modifier GC to these services.

Related issues:

Teaching physician rules vary by the type of service performed: procedures, E/M services, and time-based services.

Key points:

- The attending physician's presence during a procedure is required to bill for the procedure.
- The extent of that presence varies according to the type of surgery being performed.
- Procedures performed by a medical student or an NPP student are not billable services.
- Append modifier GC to these services.

See also: Teaching physician rules for E/M services, teaching physician rules for primary care, teaching physician rules for critical care, teaching physician rules for medical students, teaching physician rules for time-based codes.

Citation:

CMS, *Medicare Claims Processing Manual*, Pub 100-04, Chapter 12, Section 100, http://www.cms.gov/Manuals/IOM/list.asp

Telephone Calls

Definition:

In 2008, the AMA added two sets of codes describing telephone services to patients: 99441–99443 for physicians making or receiving phone calls to/from patients and 98966–98968 for Non-Physician Practitioners (NPPs) making or receiving calls to/from patients. CPT® uses the term qualified non-physician healthcare professional instead of NPP. Medicare has given these new codes a status indicator of non-covered. Most private payers do not pay for the services either.

Explanation:

Physicians and NPPs spend considerable time talking to patients on the phone. They report diagnostic results, assess new symptoms, renew prescriptions and give advice. Historically, they were not paid for these services.

Codes: 99441–99443 and 98966–98968.

Coverage: Non-covered by Medicare.

Billing and coding rules:

Physicians are often frustrated by the inability to be paid for the enormous amount of time they spend on the phone. Since the inception of RBRVS, Medicare has considered phone calls to/from patients and about patients to be part of the pre-work and post-work of another professional service. Similarly, most third-party payers denied payment for phone calls, and their contracts did not allow the practice to bill the patient for the service.

The new codes have very specific definitions and their use is restricted both before and after an E/M service. The codes may not be billed if an E/M service is scheduled within 24 hours or the first available appointment as a result of the call. They may not be reported for seven days after an E/M service.

Medicare published its regulation about phone calls in the Physician Fee Schedule in 1991.

Physician Fee Schedule Final Rule dated November 25, 1991, Vol 56, No. 227, page 59533:

> "Although CPT® has codes for telephone calls, carriers must not make separate payment for telephone calls. Medicare's policy has always been and will continue to be that telephone calls are part of the physician work in the visit or service and that payment for the visit or service encompasses

the payment for the telephone call. The work in the telephone calls is already included in the RVUs for the visit since it is part of the pre and post work of the service."

If the phone calls as described in the CPT® book are not related to an E/M service, then they can be billed to a Medicare patient. If the phone calls are related to an E/M service, they may not be billed to the patient. Although an ABN is not required for non-covered services, CMS recommends obtaining one. However, it isn't easy to obtain an ABN for a phone call prior to the phone call. Phone calls are usually unscheduled, and of course, the patient isn't there to sign an ABN.

If billing these services to Medicare patients, be sure they meet the criteria of the CPT® description, and that they are not pre-work or post-work for an E/M.

Related issues:

Care Plan Oversight is one service that allows a physician to be paid for non–face-to-face time. The anti-coagulation management codes, 99363–99364, have a status indicator of bundled, and so may not be billed to the patient with or without a modifier. Starting in 2015, CMS will also pay for chronic care management with HCPCS codes.

Key points:
- Review the billing rules carefully.
- These are time-based codes, so document time in the medical record.
- Check with your third-party payers for coverage rules, and to see if your contract allows you to bill the patient.

Citations:

CPT® Changes: An Insider's View 2008

CPT® Assistant Mar 08:6

Time-based Codes

Definition:

Many types of service are time-based, including psychiatry, physical medicine, and critical care. Therefore, the definition of some CPT® codes includes time.

Explanation:

When providing a service for which the definition of its CPT® code includes a time component, or when billing an E/M code based on time, you must document time in the medical record. You can also use time to select E/M codes if typical time is listed for that code in the CPT® book, and the visit is predominantly counseling and coordination of care. Document the total time of the visit, the fact that more than 50% of the visit was counseling and the nature of the counseling.

Codes:

Varied, including some E/M codes, discharge services, critical care, prolonged services, education services, psychiatry, and physical medicine.

Coverage: Not applicable.

Billing and coding rules:

For some services, the clinician can simply write the total time spent providing the service as the final sentence of the note, at the heading of the note, or on the form that documents the service. Physical therapists often use a form that describes the service parameters, and one of these is time. For critical care, the physician should document the total time spent in caring for the patient on a particular calendar date or during a 24-hour period. Document time in the medical record, not just on the billing record. Medicare requires start and stop time for prolonged services.

Many E/M codes can be billed using time as the determining factor for selecting the level of service. Time is the trump card when certain conditions are met, such as when more than 50% of the visit was spent in counseling or coordination of care. Here's how the CPT® book describes the content of counseling:

Counseling is discussion with patient and/or family regarding:
- Diagnostic results, impressions, recommended diagnostic studies
- Prognosis
- Risks and benefits of management

- Instructions for management
- Importance of compliance
- Risk factor reduction
- Patient and family education

Document:
- Total time for the visit
- Statement that more than 50% of the visit was counseling
- Description of the nature of the counseling

When using time to select an E/M service in the office or outpatient department, define total time as the time the clinician spends face-to-face with the patient. For hospital services, define the total time as the unit time. To bill hospital services based on time, more than 50% of the unit time must be spent in face-to-face counseling with the patient. You may not include staff time in the time spent; only the billing provider's time counts.

These definitions say, "with the patient and/or family." However, keep in mind that Medicare requires the clinician to have a face-to-face service with the beneficiary to bill for the service.

For some patients, however, the provider must spend an unusual amount of time treating and discussing their problems, above and beyond what is typical for the level of service provided. A set of add-on codes may be used with office visits, outpatient consults, and home visits (99354–99355), and a set of codes may be used with initial hospital services, subsequent hospital visits and inpatient consultations (99356–99357). These are called prolonged services codes and describe just that: a service that is prolonged beyond the usual.

These codes are a little tricky for providers. They require face-to-face direct patient contact with the billing provider, not a staff person. The prolonged service does not need to be continuous, but it must add up to 30 to 74 minutes more than the typical time for the service. That means the total time for prolonged services varies according to the base code of the service provided. Here's how the *Medicare Claims Processing Manual* describes it:

> Prolonged services codes can be billed only if the total duration of all physician direct face-to-face service (including the visit) equals or exceeds the threshold time for the evaluation and management service the physician provided (typical time plus 30 minutes). If the total duration of direct face-to-face time does not equal or exceed the threshold time for the level of evaluation and management service the physician provided, the physician may not bill for prolonged services.

Why might a service be prolonged? Sometimes, the patient is unable to understand the problem or home care instructions without extensive and repeated explanations. A discussion with the patient might involve highly emotional issues that require longer than usual physician time. Or a patient may need to have a long discussion with a provider when weighing the risks and benefits of multiple treatment options for a serious illness.

Related issues:

In the past, clinicians expressed reluctance to document time in the medical record. Most now understand when to do so, and do it. If the definition of a code is time-based, not documenting time results in no payment for the service.

Key points:

- Document time in the medical record when time is used to select the level of service.
- For E/M services in which time is the determining factor, document the total time of the visit, the fact that more than 50% was spent in counseling, and the nature of the counseling. Select your level of service based on the total time.
- For prolonged services, select the level of E/M code that you provided and documented. If your total time spent with the patient was 30 minutes more than the typical time, you may append a prolonged services code. Document the total time, and use the chart to select the appropriate code.
- Document critical care time in the note.
- Document time in the discharge summary for the second level hospital discharge service.

See also: Critical care, prolonged services code, teaching physician rules for time-based codes.

Citation:

CMS, *Medicare Claims Processing Manual*, Pub. 100-04, Chapter 12, Section 30.6.15.1, http://www.cms.gov/Manuals/IOM/list.asp

Transitional Care Management (TCM) Services

Definition:

Transitional Care Management (TCM) codes were developed in 2013 to describe a set of face-to-face and non-face-to-face services provided to medically and socially complex patients discharged from a facility to a non-facility setting.

Explanation:

CPT® describes TCM using two codes.

99495: TCM Services with the following required elements:
- Communication (direct contact, telephone, electronic) with the patient and/or caregiver within two business days of discharge
- Medical decision making of at least moderate complexity during the service period
- Face-to-face visit within 14 calendar days of discharge.

99496: TCM Services with the following required elements:
- Communication (direct contact, telephone, electronic) with the patient and/or caregiver within two business days of discharge
- Medical decision making of at least high complexity during the service period
- Face-to-face visit, within seven calendar days of discharge.

Medical practices often provide extensive non-face-to-face services during the transition from facility care to home for patients who are complex. These codes allow a practice to be paid for some of these services during the first 30 days after discharge.

Codes: 99495 and 99496

Coverage: Medicare and most commercial payers.

Billing and coding rules:

Report these codes for new or established patients being discharged from a facility to a non-facility setting. The patient must have medical or psychosocial problems that require moderate or high complexity medical decision-making during the transition and require additional support during this transition. The patient must be discharged from inpatient setting, partial hospital, observation status, or skilled nursing facility/ nursing facility to the patient's community setting, defined as home, domiciliary, rest home or assisted living. An Emergency Department visit does not meet the requirement.

The service includes and mandates all of the components listed in the CPT® description and non-face-to-face services. In two business days, the practice must have direct contact with the patient. Someone from the practice must call the patient, or have an email contact with the patient. That service could be provided by non-clinical staff, confirming the patient's appointment, making sure the patient has their discharge medication. If the patient has questions, triage the patient to a clinical staff member. Some practices have a clinical staff member make the call. Within 7 or 14 calendar dates, depending on the code and complexity of the patient, the provider must have a face-to-face service with the patient. This E/M service could be in the office, patient's home, assisted living facility, or domiciliary setting. During the 29-day period after the date of discharge, the practice must provide non-face-to-face services, such as communicating by phone with the patient and/or caregiver regarding care, communicating with home health agencies or other community caregivers, patient and/or family education and support, assessing and supporting the treatment plan, identifying community and health resources, and facilitating access to these community resources and medical care.

As of January 1, 2016, CMS stated that the TCM code (99495 or 99496) could be reported on the day of the E/M service. A practice does not have to wait until the 30-day period is over. This is a change in policy. It doesn't change the requirement that during the 30 day TCM period, the physician, non-physician practitioner or clinical staff must be providing some type of non-face-to-face service to support the patient's transition to home. This could include care coordination with other health care professionals or agencies or phone or email discussions with the patient and/or family members.

On page 132 of the 2016 Physician Fee Schedule Rule, CMS wrote "Regarding TCM services, we are adopting the commenters' suggestions that the required date of service reported on the when the face-to-face visit is completed, consistent with current policy governing the reporting of global surgery and other bundles of services under the PFS. We will revise the existing subregulatory guidance for TCM services accordingly."

Subsequent face-to-face services after the initial E/M service are separately reportable. There is no modifier to report these E/M services after the first TCM service. The discharge visit is not considered part of the TCM service and does not meet any of the TCM requirements.

The clinician should obtain and review the discharge summary; review the need for pending or follow-up diagnostic tests; interact with other healthcare professionals involved in the patient's care; provide education of patient, or family, or caregiver; establish or reestablish referrals, and assist in scheduling medical care or community care.

Some services are bundled into TCM. According to CPT® and the Centers for Medicare and Medicaid Services (CMS), these services may not be reported during the TCM period. These codes that may not be billed with the TCM codes are Care Plan Oversight (99339, 99340, 99474-99380, G0181, G0182), prolonged services without patient contact (99358, 99359), anticoagulant management (99363, 99364), medical team conferences (99366–99368), education and training (98960-98962, 99441-99443), end stage renal disease services (90951-90970), online medical evaluation (98969, 99444). Preparation of special reports (99080), analysis of data (99090, 99091), complex care coordination services (99487–99489), or medication therapy services (99605–99607) during the time period covered by the TCM codes, which is 29 days after discharge. Of course, many of the codes in the list above are not reimbursed by Medicare or most insurance companies.

	CMS	**CPT®**
Contact within two days	Two documented attempts meets requirements	Two attempts meets requirements
Other staff	"Medicare encourages practitioners to follow CPT® guidance in reporting TCM services. Medicare requires that when a practitioner bills Medicare for services and supplies commonly furnished in physician offices, the practitioner must meet the "incident to" requirements described in Chapter 15 Section 60 of the Benefit Policy Manual 100- 02." This section does not mandate require staff members who provide incident to services be licensed nurses.	"Services performed by the physician or other qualified health care professional and/ or licensed clinical staff under his or her supervision."

Related issues:

This is an instance in which non-face-to-face services are paid. The physician does not need to do all of the work. Staff members can make phone calls and provide education and referrals.

Key points:

- As of January 1, 2016, submit the claim with the TCM codes on the day of the face-to-face visit. Do not report an E/M service for that day.
- If the patient is readmitted during the TCM period and the physician continues to provide support, the group could report TCM for the first or the second admission. The physician may not report TCM services for overlapping time periods.
- Physicians, Physician Assistants (PAs), Nurse Practitioners (NPs), Clinical Nurse Midwives and Clinical Nurse Specialists may provide and report TCM. Only a clinician who can report an E/M service may report TCM.
- The patient must have moderate or high complexity medical decision-making any time during the 30-day TCM period. Use the Documentation Guidelines of complexity to assess MDM.

See also: Documentation Guidelines

Citations:

http://www.cms.gov/Medicare/Medicare-Fee-for-Service-Payment/ PhysicianFeeSched/ Downloads/FAQ-TCMS.pdf

http://www.cms.gov/Outreach-and-Education/Medicare-Learning-Network-MLN/ MLNProducts/Downloads/Transitional-Care-ManagementServicesFactSheet ICN908628.pdf

https://www.federalregister.gov/articles/2015/11/16/2015–28005/medicare-program-revisions-to-payment-policies-under-the-physician-fee-schedule-and-other-revisions

Welcome to Medicare

Definition:

The Welcome to Medicare Visit or Initial Preventive Physical Exam (IPPE) is a one-time benefit for new Medicare beneficiaries. The goal of this service is disease prevention, health promotion and education, counseling, and referral for covered preventive medicine services. Medicare beneficiaries are eligible for the service during their first twelve months on Medicare.

Explanation:

The Welcome to Medicare Visit was implemented as part of the Medicare Modernization Act passed in July of 2004. The benefit had an effective date of January 1, 2005, and changes were made in 2009. Any Medicare beneficiary who became eligible for Medicare after that date was eligible for the service within the first twelve months of his or her benefit period.

Codes:

G0402 Welcome to Medicare visit; Diagnosis, use a code from category Z00 or medical diagnosis.

G0403 EKG with interpretation and report; Diagnosis, use a code from category Z00 or medical diagnosis.

G0404 Tracing only; Diagnosis same as above.

G0405 Report only; Diagnosis same as above.

Coverage:

This is a Medicare covered service only. Other payers typically do not pay for these codes. The patient is not charged a co-pay or deductible for this service.

Billing and coding rules:

This service is not your usual preventive service, and the definition of this service does not correspond to the visit described by CPT® codes 99381–99397. It differs from the annual preventive medicine exam and has specific requirements. Here's how the Internet Only Manual from Medicare describes the components of the IPPE:

> The Initial Preventive Physical Examination (IPPE), or "Welcome to Medicare Visit," is a preventive Evaluation and Management service (E/M) that includes the following: (1) review of the individual's medical and social history with attention to modifiable risk factors for disease detection; (2) review of the individual's potential (risk factors)

for depression or other mood disorders; (3) review of the individual's functional ability and level of safety; (4) a physical examination to include measurement of the individual's height, weight, blood pressure, a visual acuity screen, and other factors as deemed appropriate by the examining physician or qualified Non-physician Practitioner (NPP); (5) performance and interpretation of an electrocardiogram (EKG) (optional as of January 1, 2009); (6) education, counseling, and referral, as deemed appropriate, based on the results of the review and evaluation services described in the previous five elements; and (7) education, counseling, and referral including a brief written plan (e.g., a checklist or alternative) provided to the individual for obtaining the appropriate screening and other preventive services, which are separately covered under Medicare Part B benefits. With patient permission, end of life planning is another component.

As of January 1, 2009, the provider must calculate the Body Mass Index (BMI) and with the patient's permission, and discuss end of life issues. This service may be performed by a physician, a nurse practitioner, a physician assistant, or a clinical nurse specialist.

The written plan should include education, counseling, and referral to any of these covered screening, immunization, or preventive services for which the patient is eligible:

- Pneumococcal, influenza and hepatitis B vaccines and their administration
- Screening mammography
- Screening pap smear and screening pelvic exams
- Prostate cancer screening services
- Colorectal cancer screening tests
- Diabetes outpatient self management training services
- Bone mass measurements
- Screening for glaucoma
- Medical nutrition therapy services for individuals with diabetes or renal disease
- Cardiovascular screening blood tests
- Diabetes screening tests

Related issues:

The provider is required to use screening tools for depression, activities of daily living (ADLs), and safety that are approved by national specialty societies. The checkout for this visit can be very time consuming because it includes referrals for many preventive medicine services.

Key points:

- Be sure to use a form or template that includes all of the required elements. It is insufficient to use most history and physical forms that are in use for other preventive medicine services.
- A staff member or a patient may complete the screening components of this exam. The clinician must review the screening information and provide counseling, education, and referrals based on it.
- Education, counseling and referral based on the assessment are required.
- A written plan is required for the preventive medicine services covered by Medicare.

See also: Preventive medicine services, wellness visits

Citations:

Medlearn Matters Web site. 2006. Available at: http://www.cms.gov/MLNMattersArticles

Medlearn Matters Number: MM3638, Release date December 22, 2004.

CMS, *Medicare Claims Processing Manual*, Pub. 100-04, Chapter 12, Section 30.6.1.1, http://www.cms.gov/Manuals/IOM/list.asp

CMS, CMS Manual System, Pub. 100-04, Transmittal 446, Change Request 3637, January 21, 2005.

CMS, CMS Manual System, Pub. 100-04, Transmittal 417, Change Request 3638, December, 22, 2004.

https://www.cms.gov/Medicare/Prevention/PrevntionGenInfo/Medicare-Preventive-Services/MPS-QuickReferenceChart-1.html#PAP

Wellness Visits: Initial and Subsequent

Definition:

The healthcare reform bill that passed in spring of 2010 (Patient Protection and Affordable Care Act) mandated coverage of annual wellness exams for Medicare patients. CMS developed two HCPCS codes to describe initial and subsequent wellness visits.

Explanation:

Medicare does not cover routine services. At its inception, it was conceived as a program that provided care for illness and injuries and routine care was specifically excluded. Over the years, Congress had added coverage for screening services to Medicare. These wellness benefits are another covered service. It joins the Welcome to Medicare visit, and is similar in scope to that service.

Codes:

G0438—Annual Wellness Visit, includes a personalized prevention plan of service (PPPS) first visit

G0439—Annual Wellness Visit, includes a personalized prevention plan of service (PPPS) subsequent visit

Coverage:

Which Medicare patients are eligible for the wellness visit? Patients who have been on Medicare for over 12 months and who have not received either a Welcome to Medicare visit or an annual wellness exam in the past 12 months. The initial wellness visit may only be provided once in a patient's lifetime, not once per physician or NPP. Patients will be eligible for the subsequent wellness visit one year after the initial service.

Patients who have been on Medicare for longer than 12 months are no longer eligible for the Welcome to Medicare visit, and are eligible for the initial wellness visit.

Billing and coding rules:

During the first 12 months of Medicare enrollment, a patient is eligible only for the Welcome to Medicare visit. Assuming the patient receives that service, the patient is eligible for the initial wellness visit one year after receiving the Welcome to Medicare visit. What does that wellness visit look like? Well, it's not your daughter's preventive medicine service. This benefit requires the following:
- Taking or updating the individual's medical and family history
- Establishing a list of all current providers and suppliers of medical care to the patient

- The physical exam requires: height, weight, Body Mass Index (BMI) calculation (or waist circumference), BP and "other routine measurements as deemed appropriate"
- Detection of any cognitive impairment that the individual may have. This may be done by direct observation, with consideration of information from medical records, patient reports, or concerns raised by family members.
- Review of the potential for depression *based on use of appropriate screening instrument* (This is also required in the Welcome to Medicare visit)
- Review of individual's functional ability and level of safety. This can be based on direct observation, or use of screening questionnaire regarding hearing impairment, ability to perform activities of daily living, fall risk and home safety. (The Welcome to Medicare visit requires screening for these issues with an accepted instrument or tool.)
- Establishment of a written screening schedule for the individual, such as a checklist for the next 5 to 10 years, as appropriate, based on recommendations of the US Preventive Services Task Force (USPSTF) and Advisory Committee of Immunizations Practices (ACIP), the individual's health status, screening history, and age-appropriate preventive services covered by Medicare,
- Establishment of a list of risk factors and conditions of which primary, secondary, or tertiary interventions are recommended or underway for the individual, including any mental health conditions or any such risk factors or conditions that have been identified through an IPPE, and a list of treatment options and their associated risks and benefits,
- Provision of personalized health advice to the individual and a referral, as appropriate, to health education or preventive counseling services or programs aimed at reducing identified risk factors and improving self-management or community-based lifestyle interventions to reduce health risks and promote self-management and wellness, including weight loss, physical activity, smoking cessation, fall prevention, and nutrition, and any other element(s) determined appropriately by the Secretary through the NCD process.

Medicare patients will be eligible for a subsequent wellness visit one year after they received the initial wellness visit. This visit requires the following:
- Updating the medical and family history.
- Updating the list of current providers or suppliers of medical care to patient.
- The physical exam required is only: weight, BP and "other routine measurements as deemed appropriate" (Height and BMI calculation are not required).

- Detection of cognitive function.
- Updating the *written* screening schedule established at initial visit.
- Updating the list of risk factors and conditions for which treatment was recommended.
- Furnishing personalized health advice and referral, as appropriate, to health education or preventive counseling programs aimed at reducing identified risk and improving self management including weight loss, smoking cessation, fall prevention and nutrition.

Will a physician be permitted to report an office visit on the same day as the wellness visit? Yes, but no part of the documentation for the Wellness Visit may be used to select the code for the problem-oriented visit.

Related issues:

Patients who receive their care from more than one physician (perhaps in two states) will present a challenge. The visits are per beneficiary, not per physician. Patients will be expecting to receive an "annual physical." This service does not correspond to the CPT® definition of a preventive medicine service. Routine care remains non-covered. If a physician practice provides an annual physical exam, as defined by CPT® codes 99381–99397, it will be denied, and the physician office may not resubmit it with the wellness visit codes.

Key points:

- Don't be confused into thinking this is an annual exam or preventive service as defined by CPT® codes. This is a "personalized prevention plan service" and will be defined by CMS with HCPCS codes.
- Visits are not defined as new or established, but as initial and subsequent.
- The initial exam is like the Welcome to Medicare visit in many ways, and both are a "once in a lifetime" benefit to patients.
- Patients who are newly enrolled in Medicare are eligible for the Welcome to Medicare visit in the first 12 months, not the initial wellness visit.
- Patients will expect to receive the service as a covered benefit.

See also: Welcome to Medicare

Citations:

Medicare Claims Processing Manual, Chapter 12 Section 30.6.1.1

http://www.cms.gov/Regulations-and-Guidance/Guidance/Manuals/Internet-Only-Manuals-IOMs.html

https://www.cms.gov/Medicare/Prevention/PrevntionGenInfo/Medicare-Preventive-Services/MPS-QuickReferenceChart-1.html#PAP

Index

CPSIA information can be obtained
at www.ICGtesting.com
Printed in the USA
BVHW010219230522
637788BV00007B/194